CU00693449

Praise for Healthy, H:

"Connie Strasheim has painstakingly knitted together a program to banish depression from your life once and for all. If you are sick and tired of being sick and tired—if you are ready for a complete system that really works, then this book is for you."

—*Dr. Kyl Smith*
Author, *Brighter Mind*

"This book is very informative and interesting. It aroused my curiosity and will catch people's attention. After you read it, you will understand what has been going on in your mind and body and have the answers to the questions that you have been asking for a long time. It has been a real blessing to read Connie's work—I wanted to keep on reading, in fact! I could not be happier for all the people that this book is going to help."

—*Shirley Strand*
 Wind of the Spirit Ministries, Inc.
Colorado Springs, Colorado
www.NewWindofTheSpirit.com

"This is an amazing book that will bring you hope and life if you suffer from depression or you know someone who does. Connie Strasheim brings a great balance to the subject, combining the spiritual, emotional and physical aspects of healing into one. Her own story is encouraging and you will come away with a plan of how to apply the principles to your life."

—*Doug Addison*
Author, speaker and encourager
InLight Connection
Dougaddison.com

"Praise be to our Great Physician for Connie's most recent work! So richly rooted in Scripture, fertile ground is laid out perfectly for the reader to begin the sowing of healing seeds. In all of my research, I believe this work to be so authentic and unique that it will literally reach people at the soul level to create a posture of hope, faith and practical application for an expected end in total healing!"

—*Dori Ginn-DocDor*! - "The Rebel Healer"
Founder, Yovel MM non-profit private foundation
Holistic Nurse, Mind-Body-Spirit Practitioner
Director of Jubilee Health & Wellness Healing
Room

"As Connie's friend and publisher for more than a decade, I have been privileged to witness firsthand her God-given ability to mine and gather complex medical information, and then present that clearly and simply in her life-changing books. But I have also witnessed a different gifting that she has: an incredible, awe-inspiring spiritual awareness and connection to our Heavenly Father. Connie's spirit-led prayers and intercession have blessed my life powerfully.

In this treasure of a book, we get to see these two giftings merge. What a tremendous asset this book is, written by a talented and meticulous researcher who also has the heart and calling of a powerful prayer warrior. I dare you to try to find this combination in any other book - you won't succeed. And so, I consider this book to be a top-shelf, first- pick resource for anyone who is struggling with depression. Depression is a very serious and debilitating state to find oneself in, and those experiencing it need only the best teachers.

Sit back, relax, and allow Connie to help heal your spirit, soul, and body, using the best tools of science along with the mighty power of our Creator."

—*Bryan Rosner*
Author, *Freedom From Lyme Disease*
Founder, BioMed Publishing Group
www.LymeBook.com

"What makes this book stand head-and-shoulders above others on this most serious subject is... Connie Strasheim. This is because Connie is not a stranger to depression. She is not an armchair philosopher, nor a lecturing psychologist. Picture her with full battle gear, on the war ground, slugging it out, day after day, with a bunch of barbaric hosts that seek to find agreement and entre into her soul and spirit. Utilizing the very tools and techniques that she writes about, she has forged daily victories in overcoming depression. This woman practices what she preaches—for real! Once you are armed with the time-tested concepts and practices outlined in this book, you can experience overcoming victory as well! This book is highly recommended even for those who do not currently suffer from depression but want to arm themselves in such a way so as to create a depression-proof life."

—*Robert Lund*
Board Certified Doctor of Natural Medicine
Author, *The Way Church Ought to Be*

Happy, Healthy and Free

Spirit-Soul-Body Solutions for Healing from Depression

By Connie Strasheim

Copyright @ January 10, 2019 by Connie Strasheim

All rights reserved. No part of this book may be copied, transmitted or stored in a database or reprinted anywhere without the express written permission of the author.

Published by Connie Strasheim
McKinney, Texas 75070
ISBN # 978-0-9961004-5-8

To learn more about Connie Strasheim's other books, visit: ConnieStrasheim.org

Disclaimer: This book is not intended as medical advice, nor to prevent, diagnose, treat or cure depression or any other disease. Instead, it is intended only to share the unofficial research and opinion of the author. It is provided for informational and educational purposes only, not as treatment instructions for depression or any other disease. Much of the book is a statement of opinion in areas where facts are controversial or do not exist. The information found herein should not be considered any more valid than any other informal opinion and should not replace the advice or care of your doctor or other qualified health professional. Be sure to check with your doctor or other own qualified health professional before doing any protocols or taking any supplements or medicines mentioned in the book, or before stopping or altering any diet, lifestyle or other therapies previously recommended to you by your health care provider. The statements in this book have not been evaluated by the United States FDA.

Dedication

To Bill Gonseaux, the love of my life, who has the biggest heart for humanity of anyone that I've ever met, and whose unwavering love for me has played a vital role in helping me to heal from a lifetime of depression. Truly the love and light of God and the Lord Jesus Christ live in you, my sweet man. Words can never express how much you have impacted my life. I am a better person because of your example and the love of God that is expressed so richly through you. Thank you—I will love you always and forever.

Acknowledgments

I would like to thank all those who took the time to review this work and provide feedback, including Bob Lund, my unofficial editor, who decorated the rough draft with lots of fun stars, smiles and other sticky notes—just to encourage me! I also want to thank my sweetheart Bill, who formatted this book and helped me to make the book brighter, stronger and more engaging.

Thanks to all of my spiritual teachers, counselors, and health practitioner friends, who have taught me so much about healing throughout the years: Joel Young, Rick Roberts, Teri Usiak, Denny Hilgers, Bill Johnson, Randy Clark, Lee Cowden, Neil Nathan, Dietrich Klinghardt, and so many others! You shine like bright stars in a world that can be very dark.

Finally, I give thanks to my God and to the Lord Jesus Christ, who gave me wisdom and insights for this book. Thank you, Abba Father, for loving me unconditionally, just as I am, and thank you Jesus, for your sacrifice that purchased my freedom: here as well as in the Hereafter. I love you and I can't wait to make my home with You in Eternity.

Contents

Foreword

In my over 25 years of serving cancer patients as an integrative cancer physician, I can say that I have seen it all. This assertion may seem to be bold at first glance, but it is made with the deepest humility and compassion in the face of the authentic tsunami of human turmoil – physical, emotional, and spiritual – I have witnessed over the years in my patients.

My initial medical training was in conventional medicine, where I was taught the three gold standard methods of treating cancer that we often irreverently refer to as "cut, burn, and poison." It was obvious to me, even back then, that these methods were simply addressing the visible symptoms, not the deeply rooted causes of the disease. Not willing to accept the limitations of conventional methods, I outlined my Seven Key Principles of Cancer Therapy™, which addressed not only the physical, but also the mental and emotional triggers of cancer as integral components of my treatment protocols.

Since then, I have treated thousands of cancer patients with integrative methods at my Hope4Cancer Treatment Centers in Mexico. I have taught my doctors to take the emotional and spiritual components of the disease as seriously as the physical. I have witnessed many "miracles" among my patients who have "magically" overcome their disease challenge. I have heard countless reports from my patients of having drastic improvement that left their exdoctors dumbfounded, calling their healing as yet another example of a "spontaneous" remission.

The causes of cancer are deeply embedded in all three layers of what make us human – the body, the soul, and the spirit. All symptoms – whether physical, emotional, or spiritual – point to an interconnected imbalance in those three layers. That is why symptoms such as depression and anxiety must be taken extremely seriously. Not just for their own impact, but for their ability to trigger and be the fulcrum of many chronic diseases.

And yet, because of its intangible nature, depression remains a deeply misunderstood, stigmatized concept – especially by those who espouse the pervasive theory of mind-body duality, which places "physical" and "mental" diseases into separate entities that are treated by their own drugs. This thinking may help in the short-term and may even be necessary in cases of severe clinical depression. However, addressing the root cause of the problem and finding true healing require us to first acknowledge the body-soul-spirit connection.

That is why this book is so important! My good friend Connie Strasheim is an incredibly gifted writer. She has deeply researched the concepts of health and well-being and their relationship to disease and has tapped into some of the world's greatest medical minds through her extensive interviews. In her many books and articles, she has given life to the human experience through her carefully minted words. She brings to the table the authority of the well-read scholar, but she keeps it real and relatable for the people she writes for – the average person, like you and me, who are looking for those implementable answers that could change our lives.

After all, she has lived it as much as she has taught it. In this work, Connie takes a deep dive into her own ocean of experiences. She goes on a bold quest to face the demons of her past, bravely sharing her personal challenges with chronic illness and depression. She is a person who, like me, has found and lived with Jesus in the center of her life and has never feared to acknowledge His role in her healing. Through her own example, she is relaying authentic hope to others who are going through the same journey. Needless to say, this personally introspective masterpiece has taken my admiration and respect for Connie to new heights.

Can I say that the need for this book has never been greater? Depression reigns as one of the world's fastest growing epidemics as it drives people to drug abuse, acute and chronic disease, and premature death. If you are battling depression, do not hesitate to pick up this book. By doing the research and walking the minefield before you, Connie has paved a path for you that could save you time and money, salvage your relationships and re-gift you your life.

You may declare, "I haven't been depressed a single day of my life!" Congratulations, but read this book anyway – you may be surprised by what you discover about yourself. Or, maybe you could gain important insight to help someone among your family or friends who is going through this struggle in their lives. I know that I, for one, have done some personal introspection of my own after reading this book and will not hesitate in recommending this book to all my patients.

Faithfully,

Antonio Jimenez, MD, ND, CNC
Chief Medical Officer, Hope4Cancer Treatment Centers

"The LORD is close to the brokenhearted and saves those who are crushed in spirit." (Psalm 34:18, NIV)

Happy, Healthy and Free

Spirit-Soul-Body Solutions for Healing
from Depression

Chapter One

Depression: A Spirit-Soul-Body Disorder

Depression is real, alive and unwell in many people. According to the World Health Organization World Mental Health (WMH) Survey Initiative, the United States ranks among the top three nations in the world for depression: nearly one-third of all its residents will battle major depression at least once during their lifetime! And, in 2013, a whopping 1 of 6 US adults reported taking psychiatric drugs for a mental health condition at least once, and 8 out of 10 had been taking them long term.[i] Yet depression is a worldwide epidemic, and the number of depressed people is likely to be even higher than what statistics suggest, since not all those who suffer from depression take medication, report having the condition, or even know that they have it. We are a world of hurting people!

What's more, people who battle depression are often treated with disdain or disbelief by society, because as an "invisible" disease, the afflicted often exhibit no obvious symptoms. They may even chalk up their sadness, hopelessness, despair, anger and other negative emotions to a psychological weakness that they should easily be able to overcome. Yet many also have physical symptoms such as pain, fatigue and insomnia, which are often misdiagnosed and attributed to other conditions.

Maybe you can relate, because you battle depression, either as a standalone condition or as a symptom of another illness—and you need better answers. Perhaps you feel angry, sad, exhausted, hopeless and helpless because you've "been there, done that" but no treatment, therapy or spiritual discipline has quelled the pain or helped you to heal.

Perhaps a well-meaning friend or family member has said to you, "You're depressed because you aren't in 'right' relationship with God," or, "You don't get out enough," or (fill in the blank)! Maybe your doctor told you that you have a chemical imbalance in your brain and you need a different anti-depressant. Or maybe your counselor told you that you're depressed because you're hanging on to childhood wounds and you need to forgive your parents. The very people and institutions from which you've sought help may have given you well-meaning but simplistic advice and solutions. Has anyone ever told you, "You *just* need to (fill in the blank), and everything will be okay?" Just pray or meditate more, or just get involved with a supportive community, or just (XYZ)?

Maybe you feel backed into a corner and are struggling to see a way out or are skeptical that you can overcome depression because you've battled it for years, and nothing that you've tried has enabled you to recover. Perhaps you are even battling depression as part of a chronic illness, and the obstacles seem too great, the journey too difficult, and your wounds too deep.

If so, I want you to know that I understand! For years, I battled severe depression caused by a neurological disease and multiple traumas over my lifetime. Tears, hopelessness and many other symptoms were my constant companions for over 15 years. But I overcame all these things, and I have good news for you—you *can* overcome depression, too, and in this book, I will tell you how!

My Story of Overcoming Depression

My struggle with depression began in early childhood. I was raised in an environment of intense fear, and my upbringing was marked by frequent verbal, emotional and physical abuse, neglect and isolation. Consequently, my nervous system was in constant overdrive, and I was often fearful, deeply insecure, lonely and sad. What's more, word curses that were spoken over me and to me daily caused me to believe that I was inherently defective, and a nuisance and burden to others. I had no concept about my true value and worth.

I have since forgiven those who hurt me, because they were simply wounded and acting out of their own unresolved pain, as we all do. Yet the effects of the abuse were profound, and the negative beliefs, thought patterns and behaviors that I adopted because of it weakened my immune system and eventually caused me to become chronically ill in my early adult years.

According to the award-winning journalist Donna Jackson Nakazawa, "Scientists are now showing in wide scale studies that long-ago childhood trauma and adversity play a significant role in how well our immune system functions in adulthood, impacting our lifelong health."[ii]

Indeed, much research has proven that repetitive abuse in childhood sets the stage for illness later in life, as the brain and rest of the body become programmed to live in fear, or "fight or flight" mode. When the body functions in this mode long term, the immune, nervous, endocrine, digestive and other systems of the body cease to function properly. This often then leads to sickness, and/or chronic depression and anxiety.

In her book, *The Last Best Cure,* Donna shares that Dr. Anastasia Rowland-Seymour, a clinician and assistant professor of internal medicine at Johns Hopkins, states that early life trauma sparks neural pathways and a pattern of hormone and inflammatory chemical cascades that impact the body at a cellular level, for decades. It sets in place an early pattern of inflammation and cellular aging that significantly increases the person's risk of developing all kinds of disease later in life.[iii] Prolonged stress then opens the door for infections, toxins and other factors to cause disease. Research has even shown that abuse and trauma alter the shape, structure and functioning of the brain,[iv] which is the master controller of all the body's systems.

I was 28 years old when I began to experience the first symptoms of illness, which included fatigue, intense back pain, brain fog, anxiety and a worsening of the depression that up until then, I hadn't really acknowledged. Then, shortly after my 30th birthday, in September 2004, I "crashed" with a myriad of other symptoms, including gastrointestinal problems, profound fatigue, chest pain, autonomic nervous system dysfunction, orthostatic hypotension (or blood pressure that dropped whenever I stood up), shortness of breath, weakness in my limbs and heart rhythm abnormalities.

The intensity of the depression also multiplied exponentially, making it now impossible to ignore. I also lost 20 pounds over six weeks. Weight loss was the only visible manifestation that something was really wrong with me, but even so, some of my friends and family didn't really believe that I was *that* sick.

After seeing 13 or 14 specialists, I was diagnosed with chronic Lyme disease, but I knew immediately in my spirit that my immune system had become weakened by a lifetime of living in fear and chaos. This had opened the door for Lyme infections and environmental toxins like mold and other pathogens to take hold and flourish in my body.

All of us are infected with pathogenic microbes and exposed to toxins, which are prolific in the environment, but some of us become more susceptible to disease and symptoms from these things, according to the amount of stressors we are exposed to, our genetics and history of trauma, among other factors.

I soon discovered that the pathogenic illness with which I'd been infected wasn't just one type of bug, but rather, multiple bacterial, parasitic and viral infections that had all been simultaneously transmitted to me through the bite of a tick. Today, Lyme disease researchers recognize that other insects, such as mosquitos, fleas or biting flies also transmit

Lyme disease, and infection can also occur from person-to-person via bodily fluids.

The infections primarily damage the nervous system and connective tissue, especially the brain, heart, blood vessels and endocrine (or hormonal) tissue. That said, no organ or system of the body is spared from their effects, so the infections and resultant immune response cause widespread damage and dysfunction throughout the body.

My battle was compounded by the fact that there were no adequate blood tests for Lyme disease, the reasons for which you can learn about in my doctor-interview books: *New Paradigms in Lyme Disease Treatment: 10 Top Doctors Reveal Healing Strategies that Work* (2016) and *Insights into Lyme Disease Treatment* (2009). Lyme is also difficult to diagnose because symptoms can mimic those of other neurological illnesses, including ALS, Parkinson's, Alzheimer's, multiple sclerosis, fibromyalgia, and myalgic encephalomyelitis (chronic fatigue syndrome), among others.

It took me a year to get diagnosed with Lyme disease, and many years to recover. Even to this day, I am not 100% healed but I can work from home, exercise, travel and function in society. Unless God miraculously heals a person from Lyme disease, which I have also seen happen, there is no cure for the disease, but it is possible to attain remission from it.

Some people become housebound, as I was for many years, or even wheelchair-bound from the disease, and the average person with Lyme has been estimated to have a level of disability equivalent to that of a person with advanced congestive heart failure. Yet many people with Lyme can look and even act relatively normal, which means that friends and family members often disbelieve that their loved ones are as sick as they say and end up not supporting them in their healing. Unlike cancer and some other severe illnesses, Lyme is an "invisible" disease, just like depression. Perhaps you can relate!

For years, I spent many thousands of dollars on treatment, once I was able to actually find and afford proper treatment, which was about six years after I got ill. Many people with invisible chronic illnesses like Lyme and depression, end up losing their homes, life savings, and even family and/or friends, because they can't work, and spend their lives in isolation due to a lack of support from loved ones, society and the medical community, who don't understand what they go through. This only adds to the depression and feelings of hopelessness that they suffer.

I've authored four books on chronic Lyme disease and talked to countless doctors as well as others who have battled Lyme, and discovered that Lyme disease, just like depression, is one of the most debilitating and costly to society. This is because insurance seldom pays for treatments, and the medical community has few answers for it, anyway. It is the fastest-growing epidemic infectious disease in the US, Canada, Western Europe and possibly worldwide, with an estimated 300,000 new cases every year in the United States alone, according to the Centers for Disease Control. This means that millions of people potentially have the disease and don't know it, because the medical community hasn't been taught how to properly diagnose and treat it, including the depression that often accompanies it.

My battle with Lyme added to the hopelessness and discouragement that I had already been feeling for years. In my weakest moments, I would rage at God and say things like, "What do you want from me? Why won't You heal me?"

I shouted at God not because I hated Him, nor because I truly believed that He wanted me to be sick. I shouted at Him because I was in agonizing pain—crushing physical, emotional and mental pain, for years. Pain will make you say things that you don't mean, then beat yourself up in condemnation for it, as voices whisper in your ear, "You are a mean, terrible person and God hates you!"

I actually loved God very much, and it always grieved me when I yelled at Him, but it also confounded me that I wasn't healed, especially when I had seen so many healing miracles before, had been used by God to heal others through prayer, and believed that God was willing and able to heal anyone who asked Him for it.

In any case, between the isolation, childhood trauma, chaos in my body from Lyme disease, financial devastation and inadequate support from loved ones, as well as my conflicts with God, I was deeply depressed. For years, things looked so dismal that I didn't know if I would ever recover my health, peace or joy again. There were even times when didn't know if I would survive.

In 2006, two years after my "crash," I became so weak that I couldn't even walk to the mailbox. During this time, I also became addicted to benzodiazepines (or sedatives) and antidepressant medications. I took them to manage the depression, as well as to sleep. Even with medication, relentless insomnia kept me from functioning for years, and when I finally decided to wean off of the drugs, I found myself face-to-face in another vicious battle for my life, as drug withdrawal symptoms added to the torturous depression that I already felt. But the good news is, with God's help, I overcame it all!

In the meantime, the battle was fierce. Well-meaning friends and family members at times seemed to wonder why I couldn't just snap out of the disease, be a little more positive, or have more faith in God for my healing. I wanted to tell them, "Tell me how you would do if your brain was inflamed, your body was riddled with pathogens and inflammation, and none of your organs worked properly? Tell me how you might do if you were so exhausted that you couldn't walk to the mailbox, and you spent your days alone, day after day, year after year, as you struggled to make ends meet?"

Yes, I was mad at the world too, and the judgments of others about my condition only fed my bitterness and resentment. What's more, some people in my church seemed to insinuate that if I just would have more faith and trust in God, I'd be okay. Maybe they were right, but I was doing the best that I could at the time. I interpreted their well-meaning words of encouragement as: "You're doing it wrong. Try harder!" Little did anyone know that I was actually sick because I was trying *too* hard; to be perfect, to do everything right, to please the whole world, to simply survive.

How many of you are depressed because you constantly feel like you're "doing it wrong?" Performance-oriented thoughts and behaviors are a major cause of depression, as I later discovered (but more on this concept later!).

In any case, chronic Lyme disease contributed greatly to the depression that I'd battled since childhood, and not only because I felt miserable 24-7, but also because it literally stole my life as I became too sick to participate in society. For many years, disability and disease kept me isolated and ruined not only my body, but also many of my relationships, as well as my career and livelihood.

When you get a chronic illness, you quickly learn that it's the rare person who has the emotional reserve to stand by you through years of relentlessly devastating symptoms and circumstances. Those friends and family members that do stick around, over time tend to tire of the battle as well and become less available to you, because they are only human and get discouraged when you don't seem to get better, year after year. Yet it often leaves you, the sufferer, without adequate physical, emotional or financial support. Again, perhaps you can relate!

Two years after I became ill, I sold my condominium because I was no longer able to work and pay my mortgage. At age 32, I moved back in with my parents for a year and a half, and then to Costa Rica for two years, where I knew that

I could rent an apartment for $400 per month and live off of my monthly $1,100 Social Security disability check and even skimpier savings.

At the same time, I managed to find energy to do the one thing that God asked me to do during those years. He said, "I want you to write."

When I first heard Him say this, I replied, baffled, "Write what?"

Before I got sick, I had been writing a fiction novel, while leading humanitarian mission trips to Latin America and working as a flight attendant for United Airlines. I had visited nearly 50 countries on six continents by age 30, and my novel had been inspired by my travels overseas. I had seen so much, and I wanted to share all that I'd learned with others. I had climbed Mt. Kilimanjaro, the highest mountain in Africa, at 19,341 feet above sea level; I had worn a burka and visited such exotic places as Yemen, Eritrea and Jordan; and I had dreams to serve God and share His love with people through overseas missions work, and through my writing.

But all of that ended abruptly when I "crashed" at age 30 and had to quit my job. I went from traveling abroad every other month and seeing hundreds of people every day in my work, to being housebound—overnight. Lyme also affected my cognition and ability to read and write, so I left the novel that I had been working on, unfinished.

Yet it was not long thereafter that God told me that He wanted me to write again. So, after praying about His request for a while, I decided to create a blog to share with others what I was learning about chronic Lyme disease, from my many hours of research on the subject, since good information was scarce and blogging didn't seem to require much brain power. Doing a blog was all the writing that I could manage for several years, until I found some brain-supportive supplements that helped me to recover my ability to think and write.

Then, while I was living in Costa Rica, God gave me the idea to write a doctor-interview book on Lyme disease, in conjunction with 13 Lyme disease specialists. At the time, there weren't many good books on Lyme disease on the market, and to my amazement, many of the doctors that I asked to participate in the book accepted my invitation. So, I wrote the book from my noisy little apartment in rainy, bustling San Jose, Costa Rica, while communicating via Skype with the 13 doctors that would become a part of it.

Writing the doctor-interview book was the first big life preserver that God threw me to rescue me out of my situation. A small publisher was excited about my idea, and the book prospered. From that, God blessed me with more part time writing jobs in medicine, which I did whenever I felt well enough to sit at the computer for a few hours. These projects, along with the charity of others, including my family, sustained me during the years that I was too sick to work full-time outside my home.

Since then, and over the past decade, I have now written, co-authored or ghostwritten 14 health-related books, most in cooperation with other integrative medical doctors, and most while battling depression, fatigue, physical pain and other symptoms.

People often ask me how I have been able to write, being that I was so sick with Lyme. I tell them that I simply did what I had to do to survive. Sometimes, that meant sitting at the computer for hours as I fought to string together two sentences or taking four ibuprofen to be able to tolerate sitting without pain or having three cups of coffee daily to keep my mind and body going. I did what I had to do and God helped me to do the seemingly impossible, amidst tears and much suffering.

Writing was how I paid my bills for nearly a decade, but during those years, I had time or energy for little else, except to do research and medical treatments, and spend some quiet time daily with God. I infrequently met up with friends or family for a meal or a movie, and social events were rare. On a few occasions, I was able to travel overseas again, (as long as I brought loads of supplements and meds with me!), and I was so thankful for those times!

In my stronger moments, and after moving back to the United States in 2010, God gave me the idea to host an online, nationwide prayer conference call group for people with Lyme disease and other chronic illnesses. I also volunteered in the healing and altar ministries at my local church, whenever I could. The sickest of the sick would show up at my prayer meetings. God sent me those who were too ill to attend church: the homeless, the suicidal, and the drug addicts. Participating in those ministries, while challenging at times, encouraged me and made my spirit soar, because I saw many people get set free from disease and depression supernaturally through my prayers. Although at times I couldn't help but ask, "What about me, God?"

Whenever I would get discouraged though, God would have me meditate on Psalm 18 in the Bible. I felt like He had written that psalm just for me, and I took great comfort in it, especially verses 1-6 and 16-19, which read:

"The Lord is my rock, my fortress and my deliverer; my God is my rock, in whom I take refuge, my shield and the horn of my salvation, my stronghold. I called to the Lord, who is worthy of praise, and I have been saved from my enemies. The cords of death entangled me; the torrents of destruction overwhelmed me. The cords of the grave coiled around me; the snares of death confronted me. In my distress I called to the Lord; I cried to my God for help.

"From his temple he heard my voice; my cry came before him, into his ears.... He reached down from on high and took hold of me; he drew me out of deep waters. He rescued me from my powerful enemy, from my foes, who were too strong for me. They confronted me in the day of my disaster, but the Lord was my support. He brought me out into a spacious place; he rescued me because he delighted in me" (Psalm 18: 1-6 and 16-19, NIV).

At times, I felt like the psalmist, drowning in despair and fighting a battle that threatened to take my life. Yet through the psalm, God comforted me and reminded me that He was in the midst of rescuing me out of the devastation of my life. He would periodically infuse me with hope and tell me that the manifestation of my healing was on the way, even if at times it didn't seem like it. In my weakness, He was strong and had come to save me, so I had nothing to fear.

I didn't always acknowledge God's hand in my life during my battle with Lyme and depression, although in hindsight I realized how over the years, He had brought resources, encouragement, situations and people into my life to help me and give me His perspective on my future, which was always more positive than mine!

And over time, I realized that I was gradually being healed, both physically and emotionally. I wanted a miracle, but God used me to do miracles in other people, at the same time that He used me to impart valuable medical knowledge to a community of people suffering from an impossible disease—and all of this encouraged me.

In my quiet times of prayer with Him, He worked on healing my heart and His words gave me strength, wisdom, encouragement, comfort and hope. I believe that I might have died without His help and would not be sitting here today to write this had He not stepped in to rescue me.

Because of my relationship with God, I am not the same person that I was 14 years ago, when I first became ill from Lyme disease. Over the years, He has enabled me to overcome incredible odds and obstacles, and in His mercy and compassion, has healed me of many afflictions.

Now, I no longer battle depression, nor am I disabled by disease, although I still have a few lingering Lyme-related symptoms. I can function in society, and I no longer cry daily for hours, as I used to, for years. I know that I am loved, and of great value and worth to God and many others, and I live daily with the knowledge that I have great purpose in the world!

What's more, my brain now functions well most of the time. I can be social with others, and I am involved in many meaningful, life-giving relationships and am no longer filled with hopelessness, fear, shame, anger, bitterness, guilt, sadness or other emotions associated with depression.

I still struggle with my emotions and thoughts on occasion, as we all do, but I am usually able to overcome any negative thoughts relatively quickly. Considering all that I've lived through, God has done a huge makeover of my life, although I'm still a work in progress. But I have learned many valuable things along the way, which have helped me to recover, and I believe that they are likely to help you, too!

I share my story not because I want you to feel sad for me. I don't like to talk about all the bad things that have happened to me because I don't want to exalt the works of darkness or focus on the negative. But I share my story in the hopes that it will encourage you that if God could rescue me out of my struggles, which were many, then why wouldn't He, or couldn't He, do the same for you?

I had no advantages that would have made my healing journey any easier than anyone else's, except for perhaps my relationship with God. I had only Him, but in the end, and as I look back over the years, I realize that He was, and is, enough.

Throughout this book, I will share with you everything that I did to heal from depression: physically, emotionally and spiritually. I discovered all of the healing tools that I share with you here while in the trenches of disease, as I sought God through years of tears, frustration and sorrow. I discovered them through many years of medical research, interviews with doctors, trial and error treatment, and most importantly, by revelation of the Holy Spirit.

Therefore, these tools aren't based on theory; but rather, the real life experience of one woman who has walked through hell and come out on the other side, thanks to the love, wisdom and support of God and the people that He sent into my life to help me, especially the love of my life, Bill Gonseaux, who is the greatest living example of God's love that I've ever encountered. I met him eight years after I became ill, at a doctor's office (he was my doctor's best friend!), and it is partly because of his unwavering love and support of me, that I am where I am at today—more peaceful, joyful, hopeful and encouraged than I've ever been, and excited about the plans that God has for my life!

As you read, I encourage you to believe that with God, all things are possible, and that He is more than willing and able to heal you, too!

Depression: A Spirit-Soul-Body Disorder

Contrary to popular belief, depression isn't usually caused by one thing; it isn't just the result of a spiritual problem, an abusive relationship, genetics, environmental toxicity, a chemical imbalance, or a soul wound. Most often, it's the result of multiple factors that affect all parts of us: spirit, soul and body. What's more, those factors are intertwined, since what happens to one part of us affects the other two.

This may be why your antidepressant hasn't been enough to get you well, or the positive affirmations that your counselor told you to recite aren't working. Which means that you can't just focus exclusively upon one aspect of healing, such as treating the biochemical causes of depression, or healing soul wounds, because such an approach is likely to be inadequate.

My personal experience, 14 years of medical research and many hours spent in prayer with God have taught me that for most people, a comprehensive approach to healing that addresses the spirit, soul and body, is best because depression is multifactorial and the result of multiple imbalances. The good news is, those imbalances can be fixed!

Yet depression carries a stigma in our society and is seen by some who don't understand it as a sign of spiritual or emotional weakness, even though it can be a real medical condition, sometimes just as, or more debilitating and devastating than cancer or heart disease. So while it can be the result of a spiritual problem, it is also caused by environmental factors like poor lifestyle choices, chronic infections and chemical toxins.

I've interviewed over 100 integrative medical doctors and many chronically ill people in my work and discovered that many of us are sick and battling depression because our environment is saturated with harmful chemical and electromagnetic pollutants, which didn't exist 100 years ago. These contaminants profoundly affect the brain and rest of the body and can cause depression. For instance, environmental toxins destroy or alter the functioning of neurons and neurotransmitters; they inflame the central nervous system, derange the hormones, damage the gut, and cause a multitude of other imbalances. This means that depression is just as much a medical condition as it is the result of emotional and spiritual factors.

Regardless of the cause of your depression, please know that you're not depressed because you are weak, haven't tried hard enough to do the right thing or "pull out of it," or are a negative person who just wants to be sick. You have a condition that is causing real chaos in your body, soul and spirit, and you can't eliminate it by simply trying harder to be positive. Positive thinking is great and noble, but most people who battle depression find that they can't just "power though" and overcome their negative thoughts by willpower alone. I know I couldn't.

What's more, if you are like I was, your problem isn't that you haven't done enough to get well. In fact, you've probably done everything that you know to do, looked under every rock for a solution, and now you're exhausted because you've tried so hard and yet...here you are.

Finally, I believe that we were created first and foremost, and above all things, for relationship with a loving God and that relationship is meant to be the most important one that we will ever have! Therefore, the closer we are to God, the better our spirit, soul and body will function in harmony with one another. For this reason, I also believe that depression *can* be caused or perpetrated by separation or estrangement from God. This doesn't mean that it's necessarily caused by something that you do wrong in your relationship with God. Rather, it is anything that hinders you from fully knowing and receiving the love of God into your heart and living out of His love.

Now, I'm not saying that if you're depressed or have other health challenges then it means that you don't have a great relationship with God or don't know His love! On the contrary, I have found that many people who have battled serious health issues are often very close to God because they know that they need Him, and have learned to rely, lean on, and trust Him.

But maybe you are like I was, and you're angry at God or you've closed off your heart to Him because you are angry or disappointed that He has seemingly allowed you to suffer so much. Maybe you don't even believe in Him, or if you do believe in Him, you wonder if He's really all that good. Maybe, like me, you've wondered, "If He *truly* loved me, then why won't He just heal me?"

If so, I want to encourage you that God is real, He sees you, He hears you, and He wants the best for you. He loves you deeply and devotedly, and He doesn't condemn you for your feelings! He understands that there are real reasons why you may struggle to believe in Him or receive His love and healing.

These can include traumatic events that may have happened to you in early life, because trauma, especially abuse, can cloud our vision of who God is and cause us to close off our hearts to Him. For instance, if you had a father who was abusive, unkind or in some other way fell short of expressing his love for you, you may associate God's behavior and emotions toward you with those of your father or other primary caregiver. Or maybe religious people in the church have judged you (notice I didn't say "spiritual" people!), and you now associate God with being harsh and judgmental, too.

But I'm here to tell you—God is not like your father, mother or any other authority figures that may have poorly represented Him. And in the following chapters, I will tell you why, as well as how you can get to know the "real" God, and/or receive His love on a deeper level.

The great news is, God wants you to be well more than you even want to be well and is more than willing and able to heal you and help you to get to know Him; it's not up to you to "get it" or get His love into your heart! He must do it for you, but He can and will, if you are open and willing to receive Him. In this book, I will share with you some tips that may help you to know God and remove any potential roadblocks to receiving His love.

On that note, all of the tools that I share here are the product of my spiritual revelation and relationship with God, many years of medical research, and personal experience of having suffered from depression, all of which led me to the strategy that I ultimately needed to overcome it. You may find that not everything I share is likely to be helpful for you or even relevant for your particular situation, but I believe that you *will* find some valuable tools that will help you along in your healing journey. My prayer is that these tools will provide you with powerful hope, encouragement, healing and ultimately... freedom from depression!

Chapter Two

Get to Know the God Who Loves You Just As You Are

Did you know that the God of the Universe is the embodiment of love? 1 John 4:16 of the Amplified Bible (AMP) states, "...God is love, and the one who abides in love abides in God, and God abides continually in him."

What is love then? 1 Corinthians 13:4-8 tells us: "Love endures with patience and serenity; love is kind and thoughtful and is not jealous or envious; love does not brag and is not proud or arrogant. It is not rude; it is not self-seeking, it is not provoked [nor overly sensitive and easily angered]; it does not take into account a wrong endured. It does not rejoice at injustice but rejoices with the truth [when right and truth prevail]. Love bears all things [regardless of what comes], believes all things [looking for the best in each one], hopes all things [remaining steadfast during difficult times], endures all things [without weakening]. Love never fails [it never fades nor ends]." This then, is God's love.

If you don't know God, let me tell you a little more about Him: He is made up of three persons: Father, Son and Holy Spirit. He is light and energy, as some of you may know Him, but He is also a Spirit with a personality and emotions, too! This God sent His Son, Jesus Christ, to earth over 2000 years ago, in the form of a man, to show us what God the

Father was like, and to die a brutal death on a cross, in order to become an atoning sacrifice for humanity's sins, in the hopes that humanity would accept His sacrifice and be reconciled to Him.

John 3:16 states, "For God so [greatly] loved and dearly prized the world, that He [even] gave His One and only begotten Son, so that whoever believes and trusts in Him [as Savior] shall not perish but have eternal life. For God did not send the Son into the world to judge and condemn the world [that is, to initiate the final judgment of the world], but that the world might be saved through Him."

Jesus' sacrifice was necessary because the Bible tells us, "all (of us) have sinned and fall short of the glory of God" (Romans 3:23). To sin means to "miss the mark." Ever since the beginning of time, we have chosen to "do" life independently of God, for the most part, which has led us to continually "miss the mark" and harm ourselves and others, and disregard our Creator, along with the precepts and guidelines that He has established for us to thrive and live a healthy, prosperous and abundant life. So we need a Savior so we can be restored and reconciled to Him, and live and thrive in all that He has created us to be and do.

Sin separates us from God, and keeps us from knowing Him here on earth, as well as from spending a wonderful Eternity with Him in Heaven. This is because God is holy and perfect and can't co-exist in Eternity with a sinful, or imperfect Creation. Therefore, God made a way for us to be reconciled to Him and to have a relationship with Him through Jesus Christ's sacrifice on the Cross.

This means that we don't have to be perfect before Him because He accepts us just as we are, once we accept Jesus as our Lord and Savior, and choose to live for and through Him, rather than out of our imperfect human nature. When we accept Jesus, God no longer sees all of our flaws or imperfections, only the perfection of Jesus Christ in us.

Jesus' death on the Cross also proved to humanity His deity, since He was resurrected from the grave three days later, proving that He had defeated death and was who He claimed to be—the Son of God. Acts 1:3 in the Bible states, "After He had suffered (and died), He also presented Himself alive to them (his disciples) by many convincing proofs, appearing to them during 40 days and speaking about the kingdom of God."

In Revelation 1:18, Jesus says, "I am the Living One; I was dead, and now look, I am alive for ever and ever! And I hold the keys of death and Hades."

What better news could there be than to know that we can be citizens of Heaven and that death is just a doorway into a wonderful life with a perfect, holy and loving God?

Jesus came back to earth and appeared to his disciples, or followers, multiple times following his death, to show them that He had in fact been resurrected. He also gave them the Holy Spirit, the third person of the Godhead, who came to live inside of them, and who would empower them to live above sin, and do the same works that Jesus did. That included sharing the love of God with others and healing them supernaturally.

Nothing has changed today. The same commission and Holy Spirit are given to all those who acknowledge Jesus' sacrifice and receive Him as their Lord and Savior. Jesus says of Him in John 15:26-27: "But when the Helper (Comforter, Advocate, Intercessor, Counselor, , Standby Strengthener) comes, whom I will send to you from the Father, that is the Spirit of Truth who comes from the Father, He will testify and bear witness about Me."

The Holy Spirit also regenerates your human spirit and makes it perfect, and it is your human spirit, in conjunction with His Spirit, that enables you to have a vibrant, fruitful relationship with God and overcome sin and even sickness. Galatians 2:20 says, "and I no longer live, but Christ lives in me. The life I now live in the body, I live by faith in the Son of God, who loved me and gave Himself for me."

When you accept the Holy Spirit, He gives you wisdom about all things, heals you, and enables you to live a supernatural, godly life. To receive Him, God only asks that you accept Jesus Christ as your Lord and Savior, and that you choose to surrender your life to Him, and love Him, others and yourself as He did, and still does! In the following chapter, I will share more with you about how the Holy Spirit heals supernaturally, and why it is God's will to heal you, too.

Here, I will share with you more about how you can be healed from depression and experience God's love, goodness, and kindness, just by being in relationship with Him. He created you, He delights in you, He adores you, and He wants to be close to you, no matter your struggles, and no matter what you have or haven't done right. Because of Jesus, He sees you as perfect!

Getting to Know God Through His Word

One of the best ways to get to know God is through His Word, or the Bible, which is a divinely inspired and anointed collection of 66 books that reveal who God is and His plan for humanity. When it is read with spiritual, rather than carnal eyes, it imparts life, health, joy and peace all to those who read it.

If you are familiar with the Bible but feel like you haven't received much from God, or have even felt condemnation or other negative emotions after reading it, ask the Holy Spirit to give you revelation to understand it: ears to hear, eyes to see, and a heart to receive what He is truly saying in the Scriptures.

This is important because the Bible is a supernatural book that can only be understood through the Spirit of God. Also, if you have a history of abuse or trauma, or don't know God, you may interpret the Bible through the filter of that trauma and misunderstand it, or simply not receive divine revelation from it. I believe that wars have been started in the name of Christianity because men read the Bible through the flawed lens of their pain or selfishness rather than according to the Spirit of God. I believe these men (and women) didn't truly know God but used religion as a means to their own selfish ends. Perhaps this meant they saw what they wanted to see in the Bible, and used it to justify their sins, rather than as a book that could free them from them!

Again though, the Bible is not like other books in that you can only truly understand it through revelation of the Spirit of God. But if you ask God to help you receive from it what He wants you to receive, He will do that. It may take some patience and persistence, but trust that He is faithful and will do it. James 1:5 says, "If any of you lacks wisdom [to guide him through a decision or circumstance], he is to ask of [our benevolent] God, who gives to everyone generously and without rebuke or blame, and it will be given to him."

Reading the Bible used to be a struggle for me before I truly understood that I didn't have to "perform" to earn God's favor and that I was pleasing to Him simply because He loved me. I read its commands like a series of rules and laws that I had to live by—or else! Later, as I came to know God, I realized that the commands were meant to be guidelines that would empower me to live a happier, healthier and more joyous, prosperous and peaceful life, and that I wasn't meant to fulfill them, or carry them out, in my own strength. Only God's Spirit in me could do that, and in any case, He wasn't going to judge me if I couldn't do everything He commanded perfectly—because nobody does, and we aren't judged by how well we perform for God anyway!

I also discovered that the Bible is a book of gradual revelation, in that not everything that you read will make sense to you the first time around. At times, when I would struggle to understand God's Word, He would tell me to focus on the Scriptures that I felt drawn to, and not worry about the ones that triggered negative feelings or which I didn't understand. I believe that those Scriptures either weren't relevant for my life in that moment, or some wound from my past was causing me to misinterpret them. At times though, God would encourage me to go deeper and pray about the meaning of a Scripture, or research it, so that I wouldn't walk away misunderstanding what He said—and in turn, misunderstand Him.

For instance, some of the Scriptures address issues that are specific and relevant for the particular culture and time in history in which they were written but specify guidelines or laws that we aren't necessarily supposed to follow today. Understanding the context of Scripture, or the Word, is important for knowing how to apply it to your life today.

Yet the Bible is a divinely inspired book that brings life, revelation, wisdom and healing to all those that read it with the intention of knowing God, and who have a heart and mind that are willing to receive. I encourage you to spend time in it daily and ask God to give you revelation to understand it, and show you the Scriptures that will bring life, healing, hope and encouragement to you.

Once He highlights those Scriptures to you, take one and spend some time with it. Meditate on it; ask God to reveal its deeper meaning to you, and then, as my wise Messianic teacher, Joel Young, Founder of For His Glory Ministries: (www.ForHisGlory.org) often said to me, "Don't just read the Scripture, but *DO* it!" Following I share with you an example if what this can look like.

One Scripture that God gave me to "do" daily for a while was Psalm 103, verses 1-5:

[1]"Bless and affectionately praise the Lord, O my soul,
And all that is [deep] within me, bless His holy name.
[2] Bless and affectionately praise the Lord, O my soul,
And do not forget any of His benefits
[3] Who forgives all your sins,
Who heals all your diseases
[4] Who redeems your life from the pit,
Who crowns you [lavishly] with loving kindness and
tender mercy
[5] Who satisfies your years with good things,
So that your youth is renewed like the [soaring] eagle."

To "do" the Scripture, I would close my eyes, and slowly speak the words contained within it, while I created a picture in my mind about what the words meant, and at the same time, performed an action with my body to demonstrate their meaning. My Messianic teacher, Joel, (who has been reading the Old Testament in Hebrew since he was five years old!) would say that doing this integrates the power of the Scripture into the body, mind, and spirit, so that all three parts of your person receive the supernatural life contained within its words!

So, for instance, to "do" Psalm 103, I would raise my hands to the sky as I envisioned Jesus' face and spoke the first two verses, which have to do with blessing and praising God. Then, I would envision Him placing His loving hand on my chest and healing me (verse 3). To acknowledge that He had forgiven all my sins, I would cross my hands over my chest and imagine Him placing His hand on top of mine (verse 3). Then, I would stoop as if I were picking something up from the ground and raising it up (verse 4- He redeems your life from the pit), and then place my hands on my head and envision Jesus crowning me with His love (He crowns you with loving kindness and tender mercy). Finally, I would picture myself as a flying eagle, my youth restored (verse 5).

Reading and meditating upon a Scripture, and speaking it aloud continually is also very powerful, but by incorporating the verses into your whole being, I believe the effect can be more profound.

If this sounds a bit odd to you, consider that experts in neuroscience such as Norman Doidge, MD, have found that you can literally "re-wire" your brain and even heal your body, by incorporating uplifting emotions, actions and words into mind-body visualization exercises. When those words are supernaturally anointed and from the Word of God, I believe the effect is even more powerful! Later, I describe in greater depth how neuroscientists have used this and similar techniques to heal people from depression and share with you a couple of brain training programs that I've found to be incredibly useful for this.

In the meantime, know that God spoke the world into existence, and that you too, can literally change your physical and mental condition, by the words you speak and focus on. Hebrews 11:3 says: "By faith [that is, with an inherent trust and enduring confidence in the power, wisdom and goodness of God] we understand that the worlds (universe, ages) were framed and created [formed, put in order and equipped for their intended purpose] by the word of God, so that what is seen was not made out of things which are visible." Words have power to create and destroy, and when you have the Holy Spirit living in you, He in you can literally change your life by the words you speak!

Get to Know God By Spending Time with Him

Meditate for a moment upon the fact that God loves you just as you are. Isn't it amazing that if you have accepted Jesus Christ as your Lord and Savior, He actually sees you as perfect? In fact, He sees you in exactly the same way as He sees Jesus! This means that you can come boldly to Him, knowing that He's excited to meet with you, hang out with you, and that He desires deeply to speak with you.

Hebrews 4:16 says, "Therefore let us [with privilege] approach the throne of grace [that is, the throne of God's gracious favor] with confidence and without fear, so that we may receive mercy and find [His amazing] grace to help in time of need [an appropriate blessing, coming just at the right moment]."

Being in relationship with God is supposed to be easy and natural, since we were created for relationship with Him, but at times I think we make it more challenging than it needs to be. We assume He's far and distant, yet His Word says, "My sheep hear My voice and listen to Me; I know them, and they follow Me." Isn't that wonderful news? He talks to us!

God speaks to *all* of us through the Bible, but He also speaks to us personally, through His Spirit. Usually, He speaks quietly to our conscious mind, as well as through other people and circumstances, dreams, and visions, although He has been known to occasionally speak audibly, too!

Have you ever wondered how you can know God personally if you only talk *to* Him but don't listen for His voice in return? While God can impart His peace or other positive emotions to you, He also likes to talk to you! So I encourage you to take a few minutes, or a half hour, or hour daily, to just sit and listen to God. Find a quiet place where you won't be disturbed: in your closet, bedroom, your car— or wherever it may be. Then invite Him to speak to you.

If you hear negative words, or are distracted, or at first don't hear anything, don't worry! With just a little practice, you'll learn to discern the voice of God. Assume that you will hear Him. Assume that He will speak to you, because He wants to. Say aloud, "I am one of God's sheep, and His sheep hear His voice!"

You'll know it's Him when the words you hear are more life giving and positive than anything that you would likely ever say to yourself! God's voice is never shaming, condemning, or negative. He may rebuke or chastise you once in a while, but always out of love, and with the goal of helping you to get to a better place. I have found the voice of God to be positive, loving, affirming and full of wisdom.

Our own biases and thoughts can get in the way of hearing God at times, but don't let that deter you from seeking Him. Over time, as you acknowledge Him continually and listen for His voice, you'll start to hear Him, and not just in your quiet time with your eyes shut and the door closed, but everywhere you go.

If you're reading this and thinking, "I've tried to know God, or I do know God, but I can't seem to hear Him or feel His love," consider whether your relationship with Him has been based on just coming to Him to ask Him for things.

Most of us actually do that, and while God wants us to bring our needs and concerns to Him, if we just do only that, it's easy for us to become hyper-focused on our problems, rather than His answers and what He might say to us to bring us out of our difficulties. Focusing on problems also tends to magnify our pain, rather than His power to deliver us, and it may be more challenging for us to hear Him and have faith in His ability to deliver us if we are more focused on the problem than upon His loving nature and ability to restore us.

I know it can be challenging to focus on anything but your pain when symptoms are severe, but I want to encourage you to look up and picture Jesus gazing lovingly into your eyes, as you meditate upon who He is, what He's done for you, and how much He loves you. You can learn more about Him in the Bible, especially by reading and studying the books of Matthew, Mark, Luke and John—and you can get to know Him personally through His Word, as well as through your quiet time with Him, and through others.

As you talk to Him, ask Him to reveal to you personally how He sees you, and what He has created you to do and be in this world. Ask Him to show you your destiny scroll, which is a scroll of your life that has been created in Heaven containing the special assignments that He has called you to fulfill, and how you can fulfill those. Ask Him what the assignment is that He has for you right now. Or, just simply ask Him to share with you those things that you need to know for today, and which will help you to encounter Him.

God deeply desires to meet all of your needs and encourages you to share your struggles and concerns with Him. 1 Peter 5:6-7 says, "Therefore humble yourselves under the mighty hand of God [set aside self-righteous pride], so that He may exalt you [to a place of honor in His service] at the appropriate time, casting all your cares [all your anxieties, all your worries, and all your concerns, once and for all] on Him, for He cares about you [with deepest affection, and watches over you very carefully]."

So, go ahead and process your challenging thoughts and emotions with Him, too—just don't let that be the *only* thing that you do in your quiet time with Him, or become the defining characteristic of your relationship with Him. This is for *your* sake and for the sake of being able to receive the greatest gift of all, which is *Him*.

God desires to help you though and wants you to pour out your heart to Him, so that He can heal it. Philippians 4:19 says, "And my God will liberally supply (fill until full) your every need according to His riches in glory in Christ Jesus."

Whenever I would get severely depressed, which for a long time was often, I would sob to God for hours, my face in the floor, toilet roll in hand. Unrelenting pain, fatigue and other symptoms will do that to you. I couldn't have held back the tears if I had wanted to, and during those times, it was as if I would completely forget about who God was, along with His promises to me. The symptoms at times were vicious, and the chemical imbalances and inflammation in my brain alone kept me from being able to "keep it together."

Even worse, I would beat myself up for being depressed. I used to think that I was weak for crying constantly, and that my tears were evidence that something was wrong with me or that I wasn't trusting God. Because if I trusted Him, wouldn't I be overjoyed? If I had the Holy Spirit living in me, shouldn't I be able to overcome this? Well, yes, but I later learned that it's a process sometimes...

For one thing, I learned that Lyme disease causes chemical imbalances that can make you wail for hours, even when you don't want to. If this describes your situation too, I want you to know that God understands, and He has a way out for you, too.

In the meantime, please know that crying isn't a sign of weakness, and your emotions, no matter how negative, aren't wrong, either: they're just a sign that something in you needs to be healed or restored. At times, tears can even be profoundly cleansing, especially when you take your tears, fears and pain to a loving God who invites you to climb into His lap and cry on His shoulder, as He gently comforts you with His presence. He did that with me, and He will do it with you, too!

Many doctors that I've interviewed for a podcast that I host for the Alternative Cancer Research Institute have found that the people who tend to get cancer are those who stuff or bury their emotions. These doctors believe that when emotions aren't processed, they can literally get buried in the body where they can cause cancer and/or other illnesses. So, it's good to bring your concerns, sorrows and struggles to God, so that He can help you to process them and give you peace.

At the same time, you will shortchange yourself if you allow your pain or problems to be the focus of your relationship with God. This is because when you do this, again, your thoughts will tend to remain upon the problem, rather than upon His presence, love and ability to help you heal. Share your suffering with Him, but don't wallow in it, as much as possible. Wallowing encourages you to live out of your soul and emotions, rather than your spirit, and also causes you to forget that you have the Author of all life living inside of you, who is more than willing and able to help you to overcome all things!

You may be thinking, *But I can't help how I feel and the pain is just too great to ignore!*

Yes, I know, and I truly understand. When you have severe chemical imbalances caused by illness or a mood disorder, you can't just will yourself to be happy and to think positive. It doesn't work, even if you choose to live out of your spirit and ignore the lying thoughts produced by your messed-up chemistry. I know, because I tried to think God's thoughts whenever my brain was inflamed and filled with neurotoxins caused by Lyme disease pathogens, and it was difficult to do on those days. So just do your best, and trust that God will take care of the rest!

Whenever I was really sick, I would also often become irritable and impatient with other people, but I knew that it was just because I felt horrible, and it wasn't who I truly was. Knowing this helped me to not feel condemned whenever I thought that I should have more positive thoughts toward others.

On that note, be careful of "should-ing" all over yourself! When you live under the tyranny of "ought" and "should" it often means that you are functioning out of a mindset of obligation, which is tied to guilt and fear, rather than love. God wants us to love and give to Him and others out of a cheerful heart, not out of compulsion. 2 Corinthians 9:7 says, "Let each one give [thoughtfully and with purpose] just as he has decided in his heart, not grudgingly or under compulsion, for God loves a cheerful giver [and delights in the one whose heart is in his gift]."

If you can't give much of yourself to God or others right now, it's okay! Living a prosperous life in Jesus Christ is about letting Him live through you and love you, not you doing something for Him, and is a process. As He loves you and imparts His life to you, you will likely then find yourself more able to give to others.

The greater the wisdom and revelation knowledge that you receive from God, the greater will be your belief in His love for you, and that His love can transform you and help you to overcome depression.

At the same time, know that your emotions and thoughts aren't necessarily an indication of your closeness with God. Trauma, illness and other factors derange the brain and it's possible to love God very much while still battling negative thoughts and emotions. So, don't judge yourself and the quality of your relationship with God by your emotions or thoughts. Fear, sadness and other negative emotions can be caused by a physiological problem as much as much as by a spiritual one.

On that note, researchers that have studied neuroplasticity, or the ability of the brain to change itself, have found that traumatic experiences, such as abuse, when repeated or prolonged, "hardwire" the brain to operate out of continual "fight or flight" mode.[v] So for instance, if you grew up in an atmosphere of fear, as I did, your brain creates fixed neural pathways based on that fear, and you literally become hardwired to think in a negative manner! So, don't blame yourself for not being able to be more positive. Your brain and body may have been trained to function in fear or negativity mode, and undoing that isn't usually as simple as reciting some affirmations or choosing to be more positive.

However, I have some exciting news for you—you can "re-wire" your brain, and even change its structure and function, but it's a bit more complex than simply choosing to be happy. Brain retraining programs, for instance, developed by neuroscience researchers, have enabled many people to overcome depression by teaching them how to calm their brain's perpetual "fight or flight" response. These programs harness the power of visualizations, positive words, body movements, and mind-body techniques to change the brain.

I have personally met many people who have been completely healed of severe, debilitating neurological conditions, including depression and Lyme disease, just by doing these programs alone. I have also found them to be one of the most important tools that God has given me in my healing journey. They require some discipline, but the benefits tend to manifest relatively quickly, which motivates people to continue them. I also believe that they provide a powerful, expeditious framework for mind renewal, for those who find it difficult to just "take their thoughts captive" (2 Corinthians 10:5)—as many depressed people do.

My two favorite programs, both of which have a high success rate and reputation for effectiveness are: Dynamic Neural Retraining and Amygdala Retraining. To learn more, see: RetrainingtheBrain.com & GuptaProgramme.com. While these programs are marketed to people with chronic fatigue syndrome (CFS), fibromyalgia and multiple chemical sensitivities (MCS), the instructors have also seen many people healed from depression, anxiety and other neurological conditions.

Meditating upon, and speaking God's truths and promises over yourself, as well as Scriptures about who He is, who you are in Him, and who He is in you, will also re-pattern and re-wire your brain, when they become dominant in your thinking and words—with the added bonus that His words are supernatural. This means that they will have an effect not just upon your body, but upon your soul and spirit, as well. That makes them more powerful than just any ole positive words.

Also, whenever you speak a word or Scripture that has the anointing of the Holy Spirit on it—in other words, God has prompted you to speak that Scripture or word—it is even more powerful, because it has supernatural power contained within it to accomplish something in that particular moment! Isaiah 55:11 says:

"So, will My (God's) word be which goes out of My
mouth;
It will not return to Me void (useless, without result),
Without accomplishing what I desire,
And without succeeding in the matter for which I sent it."

However, in order for your brain to be fully "re-wired" by the Word of God, His thoughts and words must become predominant in your daily life. That means consistently speaking His truths, and continually refusing negative thoughts and speech patterns. Of course, this can be very difficult if you battle depression, because the chemistry of your brain may be quite compromised and the neural pathways "hardwired" to focus on negative thoughts and emotions, but with God, all things are possible (Matthew 19:26).

Nonetheless, you may find that a brain-training program that incorporates the power of God's Word to be an easier approach, since, as I mentioned, these programs provide a framework for mind renewal and tools that can motivate and fast-track people who battle mental disorders into new, healthier beliefs and thoughts. The brain training programs aren't just about changing your mind or learning to think positive though; they actually heal your limbic system, or the emotional part of your brain that keeps your body stuck in "fight or flight" mode and which affects your thoughts and physical body. By healing the limbic system through a variety of mind-body tools, your brain can more easily adopt healthier thinking patterns. In turn, the chemistry of your body changes, and with that, your emotions and thought patterns.

Brain training isn't a substitute for finding wholeness through relationship with God though, since God is love and love is the ultimate healer! What's more, God empowers you to live a supernatural life according to His plans and purposes, which are above and beyond and far better than anything that you could accomplish in the natural realm.

In fact, I believe that God's Spirit and His Word can heal a person more completely than any program or medicine, but perhaps many of us don't experience healing or renewed life through it because we haven't received a true revelation of its power, so we don't implement it as much as we could into our daily lives. We don't really believe in our hearts that

God is good and that there is supernatural, life changing power in His Word and that it can and will heal us as we live it out. But there is, so I encourage you to believe it, feel it, choose to live it out—and see what happens!

In any case, the principles of neuroplasticity demonstrate scientifically how renewing your mind with God's Word can heal your brain and the rest of your body. So, whether you choose to immerse yourself in the Word of God or use a brain training program or other tool to help you along, just know that God can work in more ways than one. And, He'll meet you where you are and highlight to you those tools from which He knows you'll most benefit.

I have also found it incredibly beneficial to journal the thoughts that God gives me during my quiet time with Him, as well as any promises, words of encouragement or wisdom that He gives me through other people. That way, whenever I'm feeling down or have lost sight or perspective of who He is and His promises for my life, I can simply open up my journal and be encouraged by the things that He's shared with me.

Journaling is exciting because God will share things with you such as how much He loves you, how He sees you, what His plans and purposes for your life are, and of course, what you need to continue to do in your healing journey. He will also share with you His heart for other people and may even give you words of wisdom to pray over them. In addition, He will highlight Scriptures that are relevant for your life at that current moment. So, I encourage you to grab a pen, listen for the voice of God, and then journal any words, impressions and thoughts that He gives you.

Knowing God Through Praise and Worship

Another wonderful way to connect with God and find emotional healing through relationship with Him is by praising and worshipping Him. It's amazing the Holy Ghost "warm fuzzies," peace, joy and spiritual "downloads" of wisdom and revelation that you can receive when you simply set your heart and mind upon praising and worshipping God. This means thanking Him for His goodness, kindnesses and mercies, and all that He's done for you; meditating upon His works and exalting Him for His attributes and who He is, as He's described in the Scriptures.

For instance, Psalm 103:8-14 says, "The Lord is merciful and gracious, slow to anger and abounding in compassion and loving kindness." And Zephaniah 3:17 says, "The Lord your God is in your midst, a Warrior who saves. He will rejoice over you with joy; He will be quiet in His love [making no mention of your past sins], He will rejoice over you with shouts of joy." If you want to know God, meditate upon Scriptures like these!

I often praise and worship God to the tune of worship music, and it really helps me to open my heart and mind to Him. When you're too tired to pray, or just don't know what to pray, listening to or singing a song of praise to God while you think about Him, is a great way to connect with Him. You can also pray a Psalm or another Scripture that speaks of His goodness, loving- kindness and other attributes, or simply worship Him in your own words.

In the end, praise and worship is as much about an attitude as it is an activity. It is about centering your focus upon God and thinking loving thoughts toward Him with gratitude, reverence and awe, and allowing Him to fill your spirit as He responds to your worship.

Some of you who are reading this may find it difficult to praise and worship God when you hurt, but praising and worshipping God is powerful and beneficial, no matter how you may feel, for many reasons. First, it can help you to take the focus off of your pain and problems, as you instead set your intentions upon magnifying God and His loving and life-giving attributes. Pain has a way of screaming for your undivided attention, and your soul may clamor to be heard, but it's not always helpful to give your emotions or thoughts full rein and obey them!

Also, when you turn your face toward God, He does something wonderful, by shifting your perspective to what's possible, and pulling your mind away from all that seems impossible, as He fills you with His peace and gives you His perspective on your life. Praise and worship lift you out of the pit, not because God has given you all the answers to your life's problems, but because you are encountering His presence, which is more transformative than any answer. This is because He is the ultimate answer!

Have you ever felt angry toward God, and some part of you felt like you didn't love Him at all, yet deep down, you knew that you would never give up on your relationship with

Him, because you knew that He loved you and you loved Him? That's because your spirit always loves Him, even when your soul is pitching a fit! Our spirit and soul can be at war with one another, but it's in your best interest to give your spirit rein and go to God when you least feel like going to Him! Trust that you aren't being a hypocrite, and instead, are choosing to obey your spirit's desire to commune with Him, rather than your soul's desire to throw a pity party.

When you do this, He can then take the pain in your soul and heal it. It may not be immediate, but by going to Him and choosing to praise and worship Him through your suffering, you may find that your emotions increasingly line up with your choice to love Him. Through your praise and worship, God imparts peace, healing, revelation, and most importantly—His presence to you! So the more time you spend praising, exalting and worshipping Him, the more His love will infiltrate you, and the more the pain and traumas of the past will often automatically fade or even disappear.

Again, there may be times when you feel like you're able to do little more than cry out to God, and if so, that's okay! As much as you can though, I encourage you to seek His face and praise and worship Him with your spirit. This is for your sake, not just His. He wants to give you His best, which isn't His gifts, but who He is!

In the end, whenever you do anything that feeds your spirit, such as meditating upon and "doing" His Word, communing with Him, thanking Him, and praising and worshipping Him, your spirit thrives and is strengthened.

This is partly because when you do these things with a sincere heart, they bring to the forefront of your awareness God's love, power, goodness, kindness, patience, wisdom and other life-giving attributes.

Then, when your spirit is strong, it can take dominion over your soul and body, and heal them too, as God intended. Your spirit is the head of who you are, not the tail! The problem is, most of us tend to focus on the issues of our soul (or our mind, will and emotions) and obey the desires of our soul, but to the degree that we live out of our spirit rather than our soul is the degree to which we will overcome depression or any difficult situation, and live in alignment with God and His purposes for our lives. There's nothing wrong with healing and nurturing your soul, but when you neglect your spirit, it grows anemic from a lack of relationship with God. Further, you can only live in the fullness of the victorious life that He intends for you when your spirit works in cooperation with His Spirit to overcome depression and every other problem in your life.

Praising and worshipping God also chases away any spirits of darkness that may be trying to influence your thoughts. The Bible tells us that we have an adversary called the devil who comes to "kill, steal and destroy," us (John 10:10), which he does primarily by influencing our thoughts. But he doesn't tend to stick around when you celebrate God or worship Him, and he can't influence you when your heart and mind are set upon God. Praise and worship shift the spiritual atmosphere around and within you, so that you are more able to hear from and receive from Him.

Finally, I encourage you to praise and worship God simply and most importantly, because He commands it and is worthy of your praise and worship. No matter the difficulties that you face, I encourage you to meditate upon the fact that Jesus paid a tremendous price on the Cross— just so that you could have a relationship with Him, God the Father and Holy Spirit, here as well as in the Hereafter. He took all of your sin and sickness upon Himself (more on this in the next chapter!), so that you could be free from those things in this life and have the honor and privilege of spending the rest of your life in Eternity with Him, Father God and Holy Spirit. For this reason alone, He is worthy of your honor, praise and worship.

Nonetheless, if you're like me, you may get angry with God occasionally and even blame Him for the difficult things that have happened in your life. I have found it interesting that, during such times, I tend to forget about Jesus' sacrifice and what He did for me on the Cross—as if it weren't enough to prove that He loves me!

God is never the author of our pain or suffering, but if you are like I was, in a weak moment you might think such thoughts as, *If God really loved me, He'd remove the depression or sickness!* —Or whatever the affliction is. If you've had a lifetime of extreme hardship, it can be even more difficult at times to not wonder why He hasn't stepped in and made your life easier.

At times, when I would get mad at God and blame Him for not healing me, He would gently remind me, "I have already healed you. I healed you on the Cross-through my

Son Jesus Christ's sacrifice. Because of His death and resurrection, you have the author of all life living inside of you. You have His Spirit and He has given you the power and authority to do all things, including overcome anger, depression, disease and every attack of the enemy."

Once, He showed me a picture of a sword, lying at my feet before me. He said, "This is the sword of the Spirit, which is the Word of God. You must pick it up and use it if you want to live in victory. I gave you the power to overcome depression through Jesus' death and resurrection, and by that same power and Spirit that raised Him from the dead. That Spirit lives inside of you so that you could destroy the works of the devil, including all disease!"

I realized then that I was actually mocking Him whenever I suggested that He didn't want me to be healed, because He sent His only begotten Son Jesus to die for me, so that I could be freed from disease, and have the Holy Spirit, who overcomes all things, living inside of me. It was a tremendous price to pay for my freedom, so how could I be angry? True, my healing hadn't manifest when I wanted it to, because sometimes there is a battle in the spiritual realm to receive what Jesus died for, and hindrances that need to be removed (more on that later, too) but the fact was, He had made provision for me to be set free.

He said, "Why do you beg me to heal you, when the price that I paid through Jesus' death, to freely give you these things, was the highest price that anyone could pay for a gift to their beloved?"

Then, it was as if He was inviting me to pick up the sword and use it to come against the lies and the depression in my body and mind. During these times, I could feel His sadness that I didn't seem to know who He truly was and would immediately repent for my attitude of offense and entitlement toward Him.

God will give you everything that you need to be healed, and to live a life of freedom and prosperity of soul here on the earth. It may take time to know what you've been given; head knowledge is not the same as heart knowledge, but as you come to know Him and spend time with Him, He will reveal to you all that you need to know, and equip you with the tools and wisdom that you need to walk in freedom.

As you can see, spending time with God and getting to know Him is about so much more than just reciting a "please, sorry, thank you" list to Him daily! He wants you to cast all of your concerns upon Him because He cares for you. He wants to speak to your heart about His plans and purposes for your life, those of your loved ones, and the world. He wants to encourage you and give you wisdom. He wants to teach you about who you are in Him, and who He is in you. He wants you to praise and worship Him so that He can reveal more of Himself to you. And He wants to heal you, simply because He loves you—and He will do that, through your relationship with Him!

Forgive, forgive, forgive!

There are times when you may feel disconnected from God or struggle to hear from Him, because you are harboring feelings of anger and bitterness toward yourself, Him or other people. While God understands that these emotions are the natural outcome of being hurt by others, harboring resentment and bitterness can block the flow of His Spirit in your life and keep you from receiving all that He wants to give you. This isn't because He withholds His presence from you, but because bitterness gets in the way of you being able to receive from Him

During these times, it's important to confess any unforgiveness that you have toward yourself or others. Then repent for and renounce any negative thoughts and bitterness toward anyone that God brings to mind for you to forgive. "Repent" simply means, "to turn away from" something; in this case, the bitterness and all the negative thoughts that go along with that, and then renounce those, which means to decide to let them go, as you also let those who have harmed or offended you, "off the hook."

When you do this, it opens up your heart so that you can hear God's voice in greater measure. Forgive all those that you are angry with, even if you don't feel like it, and even if you must do it daily. As hard as forgiveness can sometimes be, God commands us to forgive others if we want to be forgiven. Even if you still feel angry as you forgive, if your desire to forgive the person that has offended you is sincere, God will take your decision and "run with it," and over time, change your emotions toward that person, even if that person is you! He only needs your decision. You may have to forgive more than once, but the most important thing is that you simply choose to do it and along with that, release any judgments that you have toward the person(s) who have hurt you. I discuss the topic of forgiveness more in depth later in this book, because it is so important for healing and restoration.

My Relationship with God Through Sickness and Depression

When I was really sick with Lyme disease, I seldom ever awakened in a good mood. Most days, I awakened feeling like a truck had run over my body. Pain, fatigue, depression and heaviness were always there to greet me. Often, the last thing I wanted to do was pray or seek God's face.

I remember a friend once asked me, incredulous, "You mean you *never* wake up feeling good?"

He didn't really believe me when I said "No." But those of you who have battled a severe chronic illness will understand. When you're sick, some days are better than others, but for some of us, there's no such thing as feeling good—ever.

In the meantime, my poor brain and the devil would torment me with thoughts such as, "You're going to die. You're never going to be well. Nobody will ever love you like this, and because you can't function, you're going to end up on the street because you can't work." And all of that within the first five minutes that I was awake! It was amazing how much junk would blaze through my head in those first moments of the day.

I knew the thoughts were partly due to my imbalanced chemistry, because once I figured out how to support my brain and body with nutrition, supplements, and other natural remedies, the battle became much easier as my mood and emotions balanced out. Yet it wasn't just a chemical problem that caused me to have tormenting thoughts; the harmful beliefs that I had adopted as a result of the early life traumas and the conditioning of my brain into a habitual "fight or flight" state, powerfully influenced my thoughts. Still other thoughts I believe were a direct result of oppression by evil spirits, which gain access to us whenever we regularly entertain lie-based thoughts and behaviors.

I had to learn to fight the battle on multiple fronts; by healing my body as much as I could with the natural resources that God had given me, while also *daily* seeking His face for wisdom and His perspective about my life. This helped me to pull out of the funk, and start my days hopeful, encouraged and grounded in His truths.

When we humble ourselves and are willing to hear what God has to say about our struggles, He gives us new hope by showing us how He sees our situation and what He intends to do to bring us out of it. And He always has a plan to do so! It's not His will for you to suffer from depression or any other malady.

Like your earthly relationships, you'll want to spend time with and invest in your relationship with God in order to know Him intimately. Going to church, reading the Bible, or even reciting rote prayers to Him doesn't necessarily create closeness. God isn't into rituals. He's not pleased by the amount of time that we spend with Him, our activities for Him, or any other thing that we do. He's pleased with us simply because we accept Jesus Christ's sacrifice on the Cross and choose to surrender our lives to Him. We can't earn His favor or His gifts. Besides, even though He gives many things abundantly and freely to us, we shortchange ourselves when we seek His gifts above Him, because knowing Him is the greatest gift there is! Seek His face, not His hand—for the greater gifts are found by gazing into His face.

I used to seek God mostly because I wanted to be healed. I wanted to know Him, of course, but I sought Him because I was so sick and tormented by fear, anxiety, hopelessness and depression. Yet God honored whatever I was able to offer Him at the time and loved me anyway. Indeed, He encourages us to come as we are; not "shape up" first and then "show up" to the party! He is our healer, but over time, I discovered that by pursuing healing and simply asking Him to make my life right, I was settling for an inferior gift.

As I've mentioned, when you're hurting, it can be really hard to look away from your pain and gaze up into the eyes of the One who loves you most. In your worst moments with depression, you may not even feel like you can utter a two-minute prayer, much less praise God.

During those times, it's okay to simply cry out to Him. He's not going to deduct points from the checklist of your life's blessings because you "did it wrong." It's for *your* benefit that you seek Him, not just His gifts. Yet He has no ill will toward you just because you decide not to praise or worship Him for a day or a week or can't seem to string together two positive thoughts in your quiet time with Him.

I believe the one thing that will keep you from intimacy from God more than anything else though, are feelings of guilt, shame and condemnation. If you feel like you're not worthy to approach the throne of God; if you live with a vague, nagging feeling like He's disappointed in you, or that you've committed some unpardonable sin, your subconscious mind will keep you from making a date with Him daily.

But His Word says, "There is no condemnation for those who are in Christ Jesus, for in Christ Jesus the law of the Spirit of life has set me free from the law of sin and death." (Romans 8:1-2). So, you can come boldly to His throne of grace!

Similarly, if you feel that He's abandoned you or let you down, or that your prayers and time with Him don't matter, you may only give Him the leftovers of your time, or you may even stop praying altogether. Or, if you base your relationship with Him upon how you feel, rather than upon the facts of who He is and what He says about you in His Word, or the Bible, you may be deterred from relationship with Him. If you don't sense His presence, or simply feel that your prayer time is dry and unproductive...you'll struggle to want to "hang out" with Him.

If any of these situations describe yours, just know that I have been there, too, and I get it. I have been separated from God and spent days away from Him at times due to having such feelings. When the pain, fatigue and depression were so intense that I could hardly pull myself from my bed, it didn't take much for me to accept a litany of lies from my brain and the devil, both of which spewed at me, "You'll never be well! Look, God promised to heal you, but it has been years now. If you just had more faith, if you just quit speaking so many negative words, He could let you out of your jail cell. But since you don't 'get it,' He can't help you. Thank you for being a contestant on 'You Too Can Be Healed'...I'm sorry to say that you've lost!" Imagine! And at times, my thoughts were even worse than that!

Paradoxically, at other times, desperation made it easy for me to seek God and receive from Him. It's sad that some of us only pursue God when we are desperate though, because He delights in being with us all the time, although He understands our frailties.

Yet at other times that the devil would convince me that my relationship with God was pointless, or I would simply choose not to spend time with Him because I felt hurt or betrayed by some negative thing that I had imagined that He was or wasn't doing. During such times, I found it difficult to pursue Him with fervency, or even at all. This was tragic because it was during those times that He could have helped me the most, and instead, I missed out on receiving His powerful, warm and loving embrace, and His words of wisdom and encouragement.

If we don't want to spend time with the One who loves us so much that He gave His one and only begotten Son for us, it really comes down to one reason alone: we are believing a lie about Him and/or our relationship with Him.

God is the kindest, most loving being in the Universe; He delights in us, He adores us, He is well-pleased with us, and is the embodiment of all love, wisdom, peace, kindness, patience, joy, compassion and all that is good and right with the universe. He is our peace and our reason for being. If we don't want to spend time with Him, then it's probably because we don't really know Him and how much He loves us, or who He has created us to be in Him, as cherished sons and daughters of the Most High God. We don't know that when He gazes at us, He sees Jesus Christ, not our shortcomings!

It's too easy for some of us, when we aren't abiding in His presence, to believe the lies of the devil and resort to the programming of our soul, or carnal minds. If you were raised in a performance-based household for instance, your soul might tell you that you have to perform for Him and be on your best behavior in order to please Him. It then becomes too much work to just "be" with Him, doesn't it?

It's so difficult for our finite minds to grasp that He truly loves us, just as we are! We can't fathom that God the Father sees us as pure and holy as His Son Jesus, and that there's absolutely nothing we can do to be more acceptable to Him. However, I believe that once you receive a true revelation of how He sees you, what He did for you on the Cross, and how much He loves you, then you'll want nothing more to spend time with Him! He'll be your favorite person to be around; the One with whom you'll desire to make time for and spend hours with, more than anyone else, no matter how busy your life gets. When people say that they don't have time to pray, what they really are saying is that God isn't that important to them, and it's probably because they haven't "tasted and seen that the Lord is good." (Psalm 34:8). Maybe they just don't know that they have been truly forgiven and reconciled to Him, or simply struggle to connect with Him because of a lie that they believe about Him.

If you have been disappointed by your relationship with God, or just feel like you don't know Him except superficially, I encourage you to please ask Him to give you spiritual eyes to see Him, ears to hear Him, and a heart to receive Him. Ask Him to put a desire for relationship with Him within you. Then know that He will work within you to change your heart and help you to know Him.

He only asks that you seek Him with all your heart. As Matthew 7:7 says, "Ask and keep on asking and it will be given to you; seek and keep on seeking and you will find; knock and keep on knocking and the door will be opened to you."

In addition, Philippians 2:13 says, "For it is [not your strength, but it is] God who is effectively at work in you, both to will and to work [that is, strengthening, energizing, and creating in you the longing and the ability to fulfill your purpose] for His good pleasure." This is a comforting word for anyone who thinks that they are responsible for making their relationship with God "work." Yes, we all have a responsibility to seek Him, but He will help us to know Him, once we set aside time to do this daily. He knows your mental blocks, and what's happened in your life that has caused you to be distant from Him, but only He and He alone can remove those hindrances, but you must choose to believe that He can, and then simply trust Him to do so.

So, go to Him as you are, jumbled emotions and all, and just relax, knowing that wherever you are at right now, it's okay. He loves you as you are. That means that when you sit down with Him and pray you don't need to judge the quality of your time with Him, the words you pray, or any other aspect of your relationship. Release and repent for any guilt, condemnation, shame, self-hatred or any other harmful emotions and beliefs that you may be hanging on to.

Just be present and focus on Him. You may want to lie on a pillow, mat, or simply kneel. Turn on some worship music and light a candle as you close your bedroom, bathroom or closet door. Then, simply focus on Him and seek His face; don't try to be anything before Him or have any expectations about the kind of experience that you think you should have with Him. In short, don't judge the quality of your time with Him; just know that He loves you and is there with you, and honors the fact that you want to spend time with Him just to get to know Him!

In Summary

Throughout this chapter, I've provided some simple guidelines for pursuing intimacy and relationship with God, but if the guidelines feel like a checklist that you have to complete in order to receive from Him, then just skip them for now! Just come to Him, without words, if you must, while knowing that it is He who enables you to even come to Him in the first place. Whoever said you always have to come to God with words or an agenda anyway? Let Him set the agenda. Remember, it is He who enables you to do all things, because when you are depressed, you might feel like you can't do anything and that alone can keep you from getting on your knees in prayer before Him.

He's here for you. You don't have to "do it all right." You don't have to conjure up certain thoughts or emotions in order to be acceptable to Him. Just come, and ask Him to reveal Himself to you, believing that He will! That's how relationship starts. Then know that He's bigger than and can overcome your mental blocks, brain fog and even the darkest of depressions, and will teach you all things. This includes how to pray, praise and worship Him, and develop a relationship with Him that goes above and beyond your pain and suffering. Simply believe, choose to trust and receive, and know that He loves you, right where you are at, in your pain, suffering and grief, and that He'll heal you, as you continually pursue Him. For as His Word says, "He heals the broken hearted and binds up their wounds" (Psalm 147:3). Amen, thank you Jesus!

Chapter Three

Receive Divine Healing Because
He Has Already Said Yes

Some churches in North America teach that it is not God's will to heal everyone, or that He no longer supernaturally heals people at all, as He once did in Biblical times. Or, they believe that miracles and divine healings do happen, but such healings are rare.

Interestingly though, and according to worldwide evangelist Randy Clark of Global Awakening, about 80% of Christian churches in underdeveloped nations believe that it is always God's will to heal, because He is no respecter of persons, and that He still heals people supernaturally on a regular basis. [vi] Consequently, more miracles happen in these parts of the world.

Of course, they happen in North America too, just not always as often. This tells you that the collective faith of a nation matters, as does individual faith. This is good news though, because if you know that God is willing and able to heal you, you may be fully healed supernaturally by His Spirit or as a byproduct of your relationship with Him.

In 2009, I attended a Lyme disease conference to listen to a bunch of Lyme-literate physicians discuss the complicated and incredibly expensive treatment regimens that are required to attain remission from chronic Lyme disease. I was dismayed as I listened to them and thought: *Who can afford to get well from this illness? And who wants to do treatment for 2-5 years—with no promises of healing at the end?* There had to be a better way!

At that time, I believed in healing miracles, but didn't really know whether God was willing and able to heal everyone, so shortly after the Lyme conference, I began to fervently seek His will about healing. I refused to believe that wellness was just for the rich who had enough resources for medical treatment. Surely God had other solutions, and not just for those with Lyme disease, but for the billions of people on earth who couldn't afford medicine for their conditions and for whom it wouldn't help, anyway.

I sought God for answers through prayer and His Word. I meditated on Scriptures that had to do with healing and read many books on the topic, including FF Bosworth's *Christ the Healer,* among others. I attended Global Awakening's four-day School of Healing and Impartation, and several healing conferences.

Then, in 2010, I started the bi-monthly nationwide prayer conference call group for people with Lyme disease. In the years that followed, and after I was more healed, I went on a few mission trips overseas to pray for the sick, as I also prayed for the people around me.

Over time, I saw many healing miracles. One of the first was a man who attended my prayer group and was completely healed of Lyme disease at one of the prayer meetings in 2010. He had been planning to go to his beach house in Costa Rica to die because he was so sick and had given up on doctors and becoming well with medicine.

A couple of weeks after the prayer meeting, he shared with me that he was feeling better than he had in years, and his lab work was completely normal. God had healed him through prayer alone! He kept in touch with me for several years after that, always to share that he continued to remain well and now wanted to do things for the Kingdom of God. Instead of living as a sick recluse in Costa Rica, he was now dedicating the later years of his life to providing resources for and helping out a large indigenous tribe in Panama.

On another occasion, I prayed for a woman who worked at my local chiropractor's office. She had been in an accident and could not turn her head or tilt her neck backward and had been in pain for years. I prayed a short prayer over her, and to her delight, she was immediately healed! God did for her what no chiropractor or doctor had been able to do up until then. Every time I visited the chiropractor after that, she reminded me of how God had healed her.

Over the following years, I witnessed God do many other healing miracles in people's bodies, souls and spirits. Not everyone was made well instantaneously, but some were, and that was enough to encourage me. Between the miracles that I saw and what I learned from my time with God, His Word and other ministers, I became convinced that it is always God's will to heal everyone, no matter who we are or how much we do or don't do, and regardless of how much we love Him.

In fact, healing is part of the Atonement, which means that when Jesus Christ died on the Cross over 2000 years ago and was resurrected, it was not just so that we could be cleansed and redeemed from sin, but also freed from disease and soul sickness, including depression. However, not all divine healing is instantaneous—sometimes, it's a process.

Many Scriptures confirm that Jesus paid for our healing at the Cross, especially Isaiah's prophecy, which is found in the book of Isaiah, Chapter 53 verses 3-6. Isaiah was a prophet who lived approximately 700 years before Jesus Christ came to earth in the form of a man, but to whom God gave more prophetic words about the coming Messiah than to any other person. Isaiah foretold many events about Jesus' life, birth, death and resurrection.

Isaiah 53:3-6 portrays what Jesus suffered on the Cross for us and what He purchased for us through His death and resurrection. Notice especially the verses that describe His promises of healing:

"He was despised and rejected by men,
A Man of sorrows and pain and acquainted with grief;
And like One from whom men hide their faces
He was despised, and we did not appreciate His worth or esteem Him."

"But [in fact] He has borne our griefs,
And He has carried our sorrows and pains
Yet we [ignorantly] assumed that He was stricken,

Struck down by God and degraded and humiliated [by
Him]."

"But He was wounded for our transgressions,
He was crushed for our wickedness [our sin, our
injustice, our wrongdoing]
The punishment [required] for our wellbeing fell on Him
And by His stripes (wounds) we are healed."

"All of us like sheep have gone astray,
We have turned, each one, to his own way
But the Lord has caused the wickedness of us all [our sin,
our injustice, our wrongdoing] To fall on Him [instead of
us]."

"Griefs" in verse three here actually means sickness,
according to the original Hebrew word, *choliy*. Also, notice
that verse five states, "by His Stripes (or wounds) we are
healed." Many scholars believe that this verse refers to
physical as well as emotional healing. This means that Jesus
bore all of your physical and mental conditions on the Cross
so that you could be freed from them while you live here on
earth, not just in the Hereafter.

Many people who have fully believed this have been
physically and emotionally healed, instantaneously, after
receiving Jesus as their Lord as Savior, or after being prayed
for. However, this always doesn't happen for everyone, for
reasons that I will share later. Chief among these is that
most of us aren't taught that healing is one of His gifts to us!

Because of this, some of us believe that when we are saved, God regenerates our spirit, but doesn't heal our soul or body. Or we might believe that He does heal our whole person, but that it's a process.

Yet, your spirit, soul and body are all deeply interconnected, which means that what affects one part of your being will affect the other two, so why would God restore just one part of you—your spirit or your emotions?

Similarly, depression is a disorder that affects all aspects of your being, not just your mind, so would it make sense if God just healed your emotions? If depression were simply an emotional problem, then maybe so, but the chemical imbalances that result from depression affect not just your emotions, but also your entire physical body.

Therefore, to be fully healed, you need to be restored not just emotionally, but also physically. Yet the greater evidence that God's desire to heal the whole person is found in the many Scriptures that prove that He is willing and able to do so. Later, I will share those Scriptures with you.

People who believe that healing was given to us as part of the Atonement and who live it out by praying in faith for others, often see God do many healing miracles in their lives and in the lives of those they pray for. I've witnessed and been used by God to heal many people myself, especially in communities, cities, countries and churches where people have been taught that healing is a gift that was freely given to us because of Jesus' sacrifice on the Cross.

I realize that some people are quite healed in their soul and still have physical problems, but sometimes, once we realize that He has purchased our healing for us at the Cross and has fully forgiven us, the rest of us gets healed, too. Regardless, if you have received Jesus Christ as your Lord and Savior, then the Holy Spirit lives inside of you, which means that you can heal others supernaturally, and you can also be healed supernaturally—either via an instantaneous miracle, or gradually. This is because you have the same power and person that did healing miracles over 2000 years ago residing within you. And if you haven't received Jesus and the Holy Spirit, don't worry, God can still heal you—just ask Him!

In any case, God gave us the Holy Spirit not only so that we could be healed, but also so that we might heal others and do the same works that Jesus did when He walked the earth. In short, we need His Spirit so that we can represent, or "re-present" Jesus to the world and walk as He did. In John 14:12, Jesus says, "I assure you and most solemnly say to you, anyone who believes in Me [as Savior] will also do the things that I do; and he will do even greater things than these [in extent and outreach], because I am going to the Father."

When Jesus speaks of greater things here, He is referring partly to miracles and healing. He commands us to heal the sick as part of our commission to share His free gift of love and salvation to every person. In Matthew 10:8, He says to His disciples, "Heal the sick, raise the dead, cleanse the lepers, cast out demons. Freely you have received, freely give." (AMP). Healing miracles are one of the tools that God uses to reveal His love and power to those who don't know

Him, but He also wants you to be well, too. The Spirit who lives within you can heal you as well as those around you!

Further, notice that in the New Testament of the Bible, Jesus always healed people whenever they asked him to. So, if He said "Yes" back then, why wouldn't He say "Yes" to any of us today? Especially since Hebrews 13:8 says, "Jesus Christ is [eternally changeless, always] the same yesterday and today and forever"? The same Jesus that did miracles over 2000 years ago is the same Jesus who resides in all those who accept Him as their Lord and Savior today. The following Scriptures on healing provide further evidence for the fact that Jesus was always willing and able to heal anyone who asked Him for it:

"And Jesus went about all the cities and villages, teaching in their synagogues and proclaiming the good news (the Gospel) of the kingdom and curing all kinds of disease and every weakness and infirmity." Matthew 9:35

"And He went throughout all Galilee, teaching in their synagogues and preaching the good news (gospel) of the kingdom, and healing every kind of disease and every kind of sickness among the people [demonstrating and revealing that He was indeed the promised Messiah]. So the news about Him spread throughout all Syria; and they brought to Him all who were sick, those suffering with various diseases and pains, those under the power of demons, and epileptics, paralytics; and He healed them. Large crowds followed Him from Galilee and the

Decapolis and Jerusalem and Judea and the other side of the Jordan." Matthew 4:23-25

"But Jesus, turning and seeing her said, "Take courage, daughter; your [personal trust and confident] faith [in Me] has made you well." And at once the woman was [completely] healed." Matthew 9:22

"When He reached the house and went in, the blind men came to Him, and Jesus said to them, 'Do you believe that I am able to do this?' They said to Him, 'Yes, Lord'" Matthew 9:28

Jesus' sacrifice was sufficient to atone for every sin, mental condition or disease that any of us would ever suffer from, including depression. If you truly believe this in your heart, then you may just find that you can be healed from depression by your faith in Him as your healer alone, or gradually, through your relationship with Him.

I believe that divine healing is God's highest and best way for any of us to be fully restored. We are healed by His power, but also because of the realization that He loves us, that we are made in His image, and are now a new creation in Him. We are healed when we know that we have been completely forgiven and are fully loved and accepted by Him. Love heals. Faith heals.

Again though, not everyone is healed right away, for reasons that we can't explain, and sometimes, for reasons that can be explained. Unfortunately, when this happens, we tend to develop a theology about God and His willingness to heal, based on what we see and experience, rather than what the Bible says.

This is sad because it causes us to disbelieve that God is willing and able to heal us, which then affects our belief in Him as our Redeemer and Restorer. We start to believe that He heals, but only sometimes, and only in His perfect timing. Which by default means that God wants only some of us to be well right now, but not others. Yet if our Heavenly Father loves all of us the same, and is no respecter of persons, does this seem true to you? It doesn't to me!

The Word of God is timeless and His truths are more real than our circumstances or what we observe or experience in the natural realm. If you believe this, then I encourage you to resist the temptation to believe that God's will is to only heal some people, sometimes, or not at all, and maybe not you!

What's more, the timing on His healing for you is always *now*. He doesn't want you to be healed at some point in the future, because that's the same as saying that He needs for you to be sick for a while, until He accomplishes some purpose in your life. Jesus never did that in the Bible. He never said, "I'd like to heal you, but I need you to suffer for a few more years so that you can learn how to be a better person."

Just as you are freed from sin the moment that you dedicate your life to Jesus Christ, so are you also given the potential to be freed from depression in that same moment, because Jesus, through the Atonement, purchased both of these things for you in the past, and it's now a done deal.

If you're thinking, "Well, I did accept Jesus Christ as my Lord and Savior, but I'm still sick and depressed," –know that it can take time for the revelation of what He purchased for you on the Cross to sink into your heart and your spirit. It can also take time for you to know Him and His love for you, and to fully understand who you are in Christ Jesus and the power that you've been given to overcome depression. It can even take time for you to believe in your heart that He wants you to be well.

There are other reasons why you may still battle depression, such as negative mental strongholds, which take time to overcome because they are rooted in lie-based beliefs that have been established in your mind over a long period of time. There are also other reasons why healing isn't always immediate, some of which I discuss later in this chapter, but none have to do with God's reluctance to heal!

The good news is, if you seek God in earnest and choose to trust Him, He will help you to receive His love and the healing that He purchased for you through Jesus' sacrifice on the Cross. Later, I will share some tools and Scriptures that can help you to understand your identity in Him and the power that He's given you by His Spirit to overcome all things, including depression.

If you've suffered for years with depression, and been prayed for numerous times by friends, family or other people, and yet not received healing, I know that it can be difficult to continue believing that God wants you to be well.

I received prayer from others hundreds of times, over many years, and it seemed like nothing changed, for a long time.

Whenever I asked God why I wasn't healed, He would tell me that He had made provision on the Cross for my healing but that I needed to believe it with my heart, not just mentally assent to the truth with my intellect. He wanted me to discover what it meant to have the "mind of Christ" (1 Corinthians 2:16) so that I would know the power and authority that I'd been given over depression and disease. He wanted me to speak the truth of His promises over my mind and body and refuse the lies of the devil. And He wanted me to know that I was worthy to be healed, because my lie-based beliefs had become stumbling blocks to me receiving that healing.

Yet I believed, at least in my mind, that His will was for me to be well, right now, not at some point in the future. I believed Him when He promised me that all of these things would be given to me by divine revelation, as I pursued relationship with Him, but that I couldn't receive them just by simply mentally agreeing with them. The revelations would only come as a byproduct of my relationship with Him and through His power working in me. With my intellect, I couldn't make myself understand and believe. My spirit had to be engaged with His Spirit, and that is how it is for all of us.

That said, I'm not saying that God requires you to be in an intimate relationship with Him in order for you to receive divine healing. He heals many people who don't know Him or even love Him, but as a general spiritual principle, healing, and especially emotional healing, happen when we are engaged in relationship with Him.

Another truth that God showed me is that our bodies receive and powerfully respond to the words that we speak, so if we constantly speak words to confirm that we're depressed or sick, and we continually claim that we are depressed and sick, then our bodies will manifest that. God can do miracles but if we don't speak words of life into our whole being on a regular basis, then it may be hard to receive or hold on to the healing that He provides, because our cells will obey our thoughts and behaviors. I really began to understand this at a profound, deep level once I studied neuroplasticity and discovered the science behind how words powerfully affect the brain's ability to change.

To illustrate the importance of words, consider Hebrews 11:3, which says, "By faith [that is, with an inherent trust and enduring confidence in the power, wisdom and goodness of God] we understand that the worlds (universe, ages) were framed and created [formed, put in order, and equipped for their intended purpose] *by the word of God, so that what is seen was not made out of things which are visible.*"

This implies that words that come from the Spirit of God are more real and carry greater power than any other spoken words in the Universe, since God literally spoke Creation into existence. Similarly, just as God spoke Creation into existence, so can our words create or destroy our health. The words of Proverbs 18:21 confirm this: "Death and life are in the power of the tongue, and those who love it and indulge it will eat its fruit and bear the consequences of their words."

The good news is, when we choose to speak His words, we release supernatural healing into our bodies!

What's more, if you have received Jesus Christ as your Lord and Savior, you have the power to make His will manifest in your body and soul, as well as in the world around you, simply by speaking His words and His thoughts, which come from His Spirit within you.

Science has also proven that words affect your body and the world around you. Words carry an energetic frequency that affects the electromagnetic field of the body and the soul. We are first and foremost energetic beings, which means that energy drives every biological reaction in our body. If you don't believe me, consider Einstein's famous equation, $E=mc^2$, which means that energy is equal to matter multiplied by the speed of light squared. All matter is composed primarily of energy!

Correspondingly, God's words carry an anointing and energetic frequencies that can heal you, while negative words are made up of frequencies that harm your cells, and consequently, your body and soul. What's truly amazing and wonderful though is that when you speak words of life and God's promises over yourself on a regular basis, the energetic frequencies embedded in those words—and perhaps even more importantly—the anointing of God's Spirit that is upon those words, will impart life to every cell of your body. Words have power, but when they come from the Holy Spirit they are infinitely more powerful.

As my Hebrew teacher Joel once said, "Three things affect the DNA of the body: light, sound and spoken words."

What's more, when the Holy Spirit speaks to you and highlights a specific word from the Bible or elsewhere that is relevant for your life at the present moment, it carries a special anointing of the Spirit upon it, which means power and provision for a situation that you are currently facing.

For example, if you are reading the Bible and a specific Scripture seems to "jump out at you" or resonate strongly with you, chances are, the Holy Spirit is highlighting that Scripture to you, because He wants to bless you or someone else with it. If it is a verse on healing, it can mean that by speaking and meditating upon that Scripture, it will bring life and restoration to your soul and body.

Also, if there's one thing that I've learned over the years, it's that even though God's answer to our healing is always "Yes," sometimes we have to contend for that healing and persevere. Spiritual laws govern the world, which means that sometimes there is a battle in the spiritual realm for us to receive and appropriate all that Jesus died for. Evil spiritual forces oppose us, and our own will can even oppose us.

God won't violate your will, so it may be useful for you to ask Him whether you truly want to be well, or if there is some fractured or broken part of you that is not in cooperation and agreement with Him for your healing. If not, you can ask Him to remove or heal whatever may be keeping you from receiving the abundant life that He has for you.

If you feel that you don't have faith for healing, because you've prayed to God for healing for years, or you've received prayer from other people hundreds of times and are weary, just know that this doesn't mean that you can't be healed or that God doesn't want to heal you.

In 2012, I attended a conference in which an evangelist shared his wife's testimony of healing from fibromyalgia. She had battled the condition for seven years, and he had prayed over her numerous times, as had many other people, but for years, there had been no change in her condition.

Then one day, someone prayed over her and she was made completely well! Confused, the evangelist asked Jesus why she hadn't been healed, or why his and others' prayers hadn't seemed to make a difference up until then. God revealed to him that their prayers *had* been making a difference, and that in the spiritual realm, every prayer that had been prayed over his wife, had brought his wife one step closer to health, until finally, the last prayer shattered whatever rock of resistance there had been against her in the spiritual realm. When this happened, she was healed.

This should encourage you that there is hope for you, too! Anyway, you don't have to have faith in your faith. Have faith in Jesus and ask Him to remove any roadblocks, such as unbelief. I've found that belief doesn't come by striving to have faith anyway, or even by reciting Scriptures on healing, but simply by entering into God's presence, spending time listening to Him, resting, and receiving His love. Faith is a byproduct of relationship with God, not the result of a cookie-cutter formula of steps designed to produce a certain outcome!

I believe that one mistake some of us make when we aren't healed immediately through prayer is to look at where we are falling short in our relationship with God. We then admonish ourselves to do something differently, such as recite more healing Scriptures. Without love, this can easily become a game in striving, and become just another way that we perform for God or try to make spiritual laws work.

But what if we just need to spend time with God our Father and in His Word, and let Him work His love and faith into us? Romans 10:17 says, "So faith comes from hearing [what is told], and what is heard comes by the [preaching of the] message concerning Christ." Notice it doesn't say faith comes by hearing the Word of God, but rather, *hearing* comes by the Word. That means that the Word, which is both the Bible and Jesus (Jesus is the living Word), impart to us the ability to hear His truths and receive them. When we study the Scriptures, it shouldn't just be with the goal of getting the meaning of those verses into our heart, but rather, with the goal of having His *life* imparted to us. Believing, along with relationship with God and allowing His Word to impart life to us, produces healing.

If you have felt challenged in knowing deeply the love of God, I encourage you to simply decide to believe and trust that He will help you, even if you've been battling depression for years. Then do nothing else but wait on Him. I've found that it's easy to make excuses not to trust God, and to believe my circumstances above what He has said to me personally or through His Word.

At the same, know that if you have accepted Jesus as your Lord and Savior, then this means that He has regenerated your spirit and made it perfect, and you now have the power and ability to turn away from any thoughts of unbelief, which come from your soul. Instead, you can simply say, "I choose to trust in and believe You." You can do this, even if right now, your feelings don't line up with your choice, and even if you must say it daily until it becomes a part of your reality.

With all that said, and as I mentioned earlier, God often heals those who don't know or even believe in Him, because He's a loving God, but also because He desires to draw all people to Himself and reveal Himself to them. He even heals those who are angry with Him, so while having faith and a strong relationship with God—if prerequisites for living a victorious life in Christ—are not required for Him to heal anyone.

At the same time, meditating upon, and speaking Scriptures that have to do with God's love and healing can spark faith for healing in your heart. Belief can become the outcome of continually affirming the truth in your heart and with your words.

Further, God promises that no matter how we feel, His Word doesn't return to Him void (Isaiah 55:11), which means that whatever words you speak that are from the Holy Spirit, will be anointed and release restorative power into your life.

Of course, there is no formula for healing. Just know that God heals in a variety of ways, and it's not up to you to figure out how He wants to heal you—just believe that He will!

In my 2011 book, *Healing Chronic Illness; By His Spirit, Through His Resources,* I write that some ministers have found that there are certain issues that seem to hinder some people from receiving divine healing, and which may need to be resolved so that they can better receive from God. Following is a brief explanation of a few of these.

I share the following with the caveat that there are no Scriptures that directly state that any of the factors mentioned here are a hindrance to healing and the cause of soul sickness, although some Scriptures infer that they may be. For instance, the Bible doesn't directly state that unhealthy relationships will make your soul and body sick, but it does say things like, "Bad company corrupts good morals" (1 Cor. 15:33).

Therefore, if you think that your character or morals are being corrupted by an abusive or ungodly relationship in your life then you may begin speaking negative words over yourself or others, which can in turn affect your body. This is because the Word also says, "Death and life are in the power of the tongue, and those who love it and indulge it will eat its fruit and bear the consequences of their words" (Proverbs 18:21).

As another example, the Bible doesn't state that eating junk food will make you sick, but it does describe the kind of food that God intended for our bodies to thrive on. In Genesis 1:29, He says, "Behold, I have given you every plant yielding seed that is on the face of all the earth, and every tree with seed in its fruit. You shall have them for food." That means things like fruits, vegetables, nuts and seeds.

Later, after the fall, God also allowed man to eat animal flesh (Genesis 9:3) and indeed, scientific studies have found that vegetables, fruit and animal protein are generally healthy for most of us and tend to promote a balanced mood and healthy body.

Foods that have been adulterated and manipulated by man and which are enriched with chemicals and sugar, can affect your mind and body. If you continually test God by eating things that are harmful to your body, I believe that it can be difficult for you to heal or stay well. I describe the major role that food can play in healing from depression, later in this book.

Other factors that *may* influence healing, based on some ministers' experiences include:

- Feeling unworthy to be healed
- Nurturing unforgiveness toward yourself, God or others
- Having subconscious motivations for wanting to remain depressed or sick
- Not believing or knowing that it's God's will for you to be well
- Not caring for God's temple (your body)
- Remaining in abusive relationships that make your soul sick
- Actions and words of unbelief, which can work against faith

- Fixating on symptoms and speaking negative words over yourself
- Believing that God needs for you to be depressed or sick to teach you a lesson
- Generational curses

Unforgiveness can be a major perpetuating cause of depression and a hindrance to healing, since it causes emotions such as resentment, bitterness and anger to build up inside of you, and negative thoughts to poison your cells. It has sometimes been said that depression is anger turned inward toward oneself, so I encourage you to check your heart for any bitterness and judgments against yourself, God and others, and then ask Him to help you to release those things.

Also, God says that He will not forgive us if we don't forgive others. For instance, Mark 11: 25-26 states, "Whenever you stand praying, if you have anything against anyone, forgive him [drop the issue, let it go], so that your Father who is in heaven will also forgive you your transgressions and wrongdoings [against Him and others]. But if you do not forgive, neither will your Father in Heaven forgive your transgressions."

Another potential hindrance to healing may be when we don't truly desire to be well, either consciously or subconsciously. A lack of desire to be healed can be the result of many things, such as feeling unworthy of health or a happy life. In John 5:6, Jesus asked the man at the sheep gate in Jerusalem. "Do you want to be healed?" He may have been suggesting that the man was sick because some part of Him didn't want to be well, and that the man needed to ponder and reconcile this before Jesus could heal him.

I believe that while nobody in their heart ever truly wants to be depressed or sick, you may want to consider whether some part of you is subconsciously or unconsciously seeking for your needs to be met through the depression. If so, this would mean that your will is divided. This may be especially true if you have a history of trauma or abuse, and are afraid, for example, that being healed and out and about in the world will cause you to be hurt or rejected in some way. Depression may serve as a protective mechanism for the broken part of you that hasn't received God's healing grace, to remain isolated. If that's true, know that God can heal even that fear, or whatever harmful belief may be holding you back and keeping you from receiving the fullness of His healing.

Have you ever heard anyone say, "Oh, So-and-So isn't healed because he or she just wants to be sick?" I have, and it has always rubbed me the wrong way. This is because I believe that deep down, nobody truly wants to be depressed or sick, even if there are unhealed parts of a person's soul that may not be in full agreement with their spirit man for total healing. Perhaps the question should instead be, "Why doesn't some part of me (or another person) want to be well, and how can we pray for God to heal that?" Never just give up on someone and assume they want to stay where they are!

In the end, if you feel that something is hindering your healing, rather than make a laundry list of all the potential roadblocks that you think you need to ask God to remove— because this can easily thrust you into a performance-based mentality of having to "figure it out" or "do it all right" –I recommend simply asking the Holy Spirit how you can cooperate with Him for your healing. That's it. I don't believe He will make it complicated. He might just tell you something like, "You need to forgive your brother" or "Stop eating donuts," –because sugar inflames your brain! Or He might say, "Just learn to relax and trust Me," which is probably the most challenging thing for any of us to do, and yet the simplest and most powerful! Or, He might tell you that He needs to help you stop poisoning your cells with negative thoughts and words, and that this is a process that will take some time.

You may think that God expects you to make radical changes to your life, and check off fifteen "to-do" boxes before He can heal you, but if you have to fulfill a hundred requirements in order to receive His healing, then what was the purpose of Jesus Christ's sacrifice on the Cross, which atoned for every physical, spiritual and emotional problem that you would ever have? You can't earn His healing, because it is a gift.

At the same time, I believe that He may ask you to do a few things to appropriate and receive the healing that He died for. (But remember, you have His Spirit to help you!) This includes things like choosing to trust Him or thank Him for your healing. Yet ironically, I think that some of us don't even follow even the simplest of His commands and we then blame Him, because we think that He has made it so hard for us to be well. But what if you just need to believe Him and do those few simple things that He's asked you to do?

Remember, the devil will lie to you and tell you things like, "You've done everything to get well and it hasn't worked!" But the truth is—and I don't say this in condemnation, because we have all been tricked by this one—have you done the one or two things that He's asked of you? Have you truly chosen to trust Him, day by day, with your whole heart, and thanked Him daily for your healing? Have you done that as diligently as you take your vitamins and anti-depressant drugs? There is great power in simply expressing gratitude to God, and in choosing to trust and believe Him, moment by moment.

Hoping that you'll be healed isn't the same as trusting God. When you can say in the midst of your suffering, "Lord, I believe that you are healing me," and you believe it in your heart, that is trust. But even if you don't feel in your emotions that you trust or believe Him, if you continually affirm that you do, over time, this will build your belief in Him to take care of you.

That said you don't need to recite Scriptures to convince God to heal you. You don't win "God points" for doing the right thing, but when you continually speak and meditate upon the truth, you end up convincing *yourself* and your brain, which has been programmed with negativity and lies, that He is at work releasing blessing and healing on your behalf. As you affirm His goodness, love and other positive attributes, and express gratitude for what He's done for you because of Jesus' work on the Cross, over time, your brain will create new, healthier neural pathways, and you'll find your soul and body lining up with the truth. As this happens, the powers of darkness that lie to you daily will leave!

Your model for healing is Jesus, and He didn't complicate things. The words that He used to heal others were always simple and straightforward. At the same time, Scripture tells us or suggests that things like renewing your mind daily with the truth, forgiving others, and taking care of the temple that is your body, among other things—will foster and create fertile ground within you for healing.

But again, please don't feel like you have to figure it all out. Otherwise, that would mean that your healing is all up to you, and God is simply the genie that releases your blessing once you "do it all right"—but that's not who He is or what He promised. Rather, He will show you if there's anything that you need to do to cooperate with Him for your healing, and whatever it is that He asks you to do, He will enable you to do. He might just say, "Believe in Me and trust Me!"

Besides, God knows that depression can create apathy and a lack of desire to meditate on Scripture or pray, so trust that He knows your need and will help you to break free from the blackness and the bleakness, despite your weaknesses. Trust Him to do all things through you. He says, "My grace is sufficient for you, for my power is made perfect in weakness." (2 Cor. 12:9).

Consider too that just being in relationship with Him alone can heal you. When you know that you are truly loved, depression starts to fade, because love heals. Put simply, you heal when you abide in Him.

If you are still worried that you don't believe that you don't have enough faith to be healed, consider that Jesus raised Lazarus from the dead. How much belief do you think that Lazarus had? Probably not much, considering that he wasn't even alive! God can do anything. You need to know that He's bigger than your roadblocks, fears and wounds, and even your unbelief. There's a difference between simply cooperating with Him for your healing and thinking that you have to do everything right and do it all yourself. The latter is a sure recipe for depression so don't even "go" there! Trust Him who can show you all things and do all things through you.

Todd White, an evangelist and Founder of the ministry Lifestyle Christianity, was miraculously healed in body, soul and spirit after 22 years of drug addiction. He has prayed over thousands of people and contends that He has seen many people get healed, even when they didn't believe in healing, were atheists, or rebellious and angry toward God.

I'm not suggesting that you should have a "whatever" attitude toward God, but I share this just so you know that receiving God's healing doesn't require you to be perfectly obedient or have a perfect attitude, even though as a general principle, obedience creates fertile ground for healing to occur. This should be further incentive for you to not feel like you need to do everything right. At the same time, recognize that if you haven't been healed, there is a reason, and it's certainly worthwhile to ask Holy Spirit what you might do to receive in greater measure, bearing in mind that just because you haven't been instantaneously healed, it doesn't mean that it's your fault or because you've done something wrong.

God is no respecter of persons, and while we don't know why some people get healed instantly, while others wait longer for their healing, I encourage you to persevere and simply choose to believe God and His Word above what you witness with your eyes or feel in your body; no matter how long you must pray, and no matter how long you've waited to be healed. Let Jesus' example be your witness.

I encourage you to believe that God wants you to be healed from depression, not because of who you are or what you do or don't do, but just because His Word says so. He delights in you and loves you, infinitely and beyond measure!

Don't create a theology about His will for your life based upon your personal experience or that of others. Decide to believe only Him and His Word, which is the final, authoritative truth that transcends circumstances or what you see with your eyes or experience in your body and soul.

Again, I know how hard it can be to believe God for healing if some part of you believes that He doesn't want you to be well, or that His healing is random, so I encourage you to do further study and research on the topic of divine healing, as you seek the face of God for further revelation, so that you know that you know what you believe.

I've prayed for the sick in several foreign countries, including Colombia, Cuba and Costa Rica, and witnessed God miraculously heal many people that I've prayed for, and in some situations, nearly everyone. I've also seen God supernaturally heal people in the United States, but because fewer people here believe in divine healing than in many underdeveloped nations, I've not witnessed as many healings here. However, if we choose to believe, I think we will one day see as many people getting healed in North America as we do down south and in other parts of the world.

Some people propose that God allows depression or sickness to teach us a lesson. Having been sick for many years, I can tell you beyond a shadow of a doubt that God does use illness for good. Had I not gotten Lyme disease or suffered from depression, I might not have pursued God so fervently or realized my need for Him. I might not have set healthier boundaries in my relationships, sought out a more life-giving lifestyle, or learned to maintain a healthy diet, all of which have been essential for my recovery. I might not have had such deep empathy and compassion for others who battle depression or neurological disease. I might not have even been able to write this book! Yet I don't believe that God allowed the depression and disease so that I would do these things. He could have showed me a better way, but He used what I went through for His good and His glory. As His Word says, "All things work together for the good for those who love Him, who have been called according to His purpose." (Romans 8:28)

What's more, some of the best ministers I know have suffered great illnesses and tragedy and tend to have great compassion and understanding toward others who have endured similar things because they have "been there, suffered that." Hebrews 4:15 says of Jesus: "For we do not have a High Priest who is unable to sympathize and understand our weaknesses and temptations, but One who has been tempted [knowing exactly how it feels to be human] in every respect as we are, yet without [committing any] sin."

Jesus empathizes with us, because of what He suffered on earth as a man. He "gets it," because He's been there, too. In fact, He suffered much more on earth than any of us ever will, because He took the entire weight of the world's sin upon Himself when He went to the Cross.

Nonetheless, the fact that God uses our suffering for good doesn't mean that He authors or endorses depression or any other disease. There's a difference between using the circumstances of depression for good, and purposely afflicting someone with it. John 10:10 says, "The thief comes only in order to steal and kill and destroy. I came that they may have and enjoy life, and have it in abundance [to the full, till it overflows]."

Depression involves the destruction of the mind, body and spirit, so how could that be from God? Besides which, God has given you weapons with which fight it. Why would He do that if He wanted you to be sick or depressed in the first place? Why would he sacrifice His only begotten Son for your healing, only to turn around and give you depression? The answer is, He doesn't!

Bill Johnson, pastor of Bethel church, which is known worldwide for its healing miracles, once emphatically stated a simple truth in a school of supernatural healing that I attended, a truth that seems so obvious, but which many of us seem to easily forget: "God is good. The devil is bad." He reminded us, his students, that the first century church believed in divine healing as an essential part of the gospel. Yet today, many American Christians believe that the devil heals, and that God gives disease to make us better Christians! Some of us regard healing miracles with skepticism and as witchcraft, rather than a valid manifestation of God's presence and love toward us.

My own experience seems to bear witness to this. In 2015 I went to Medellin, Colombia on a mission trip. While there, I prayed over some of the staff at a local ministry, along with some members of a US church who had also come to Colombia to minister to the local people.

One day, the Spirit fell so heavily upon the staff while I was praying over them, that they all fell to the ground, and their faces became flecked with specks of gold! One woman's ankle was completely healed.

I was delighted and in awe of God's touch upon the local church, but the pastor of the US church, who had never seen such signs and wonders, was apparently intimidated by the manifestation of the Spirit and the woman's healing, because he later told the head of the local ministry that he didn't want me ministering with his church members that were visiting from the US. I was then excluded from the remainder of the activities, because the US church financially supported the local ministry, and I suppose the local ministry didn't want to lose their support. I was saddened, but then realized that somebody should have explained to the pastor of the US church beforehand why God still does signs and wonders and heals people today.

None of us walks perfectly in the Spirit or has received the full revelation of God's love and knowledge about healing. My healing from Lyme and depression wasn't instantaneous, but some people's is. There are spiritual forces that come against us, and as I mentioned, our own will can oppose us. For these and probably other reasons, God also uses resources in the natural realm to heal us, including medicine. We in the US have access to more medicine than people in third world countries, so perhaps it's easier for us to put our hope in medicine than in God, although in the end, our hope should always be in Him, regardless of what method He uses to heal us, or how.

In any case, God has provided more than enough evidence through the Scriptures that He is willing and able to heal everyone, and if there is one truth that I hope you'll embrace in this entire chapter, it's this!

Later in this book, I also describe some of the tools in medicine that God gave me to heal from depression, and which I believe may help you, too. Medicine was a godsend to me because it helped to tame my emotions, function, and focus in prayer. It is your spirit that communicates with God, but your brain and mind work in cooperation with your spirit, so you may find it important to support your brain and the rest of your body, too. Medicine also helped me to get up and get going and minister to others, when I otherwise would not have been able to. It also removed many of the biochemical factors that were contributing to my depression, so I highly recommend medicine, especially natural medicine, to anyone who is struggling to receive healing through faith in God alone. At the same time, I encourage you to be led by the Spirit in all things. Don't do something just because I suggest it, but only because the Spirit tells you that it's what you need.

At this point, if you still aren't yet convinced that depression or disease aren't God's plan for your life, and/or you are still wondering if He wants you to be well, consider all of the additional reasons why sickness isn't His will:

(Note: The following excerpts are taken from my 2010 book, *Healing Chronic Illness: By His Spirit, Through His Resources.*)

1) God didn't design us for depression or disease. He didn't create depressed or sick people. He made us to be healthy and whole, as reflected in the image of Adam and Eve in the Garden of Eden before sin came into the world.

2) Disease and depression are never called a blessing in the Bible. I can't find a single instance in the Bible where God called disease a blessing. Can you?

3) One of His names is Jehovah-Rapha, which means, "I am the Lord that heals you." "Jehovah" means "the Eternal One" and "Rapha" is the Hebrew word for "heal." Did you know that God has a number of names in Hebrew, according to His attributes? The Lord That Heals is one of them.

4) Depression and disease limit our ability to go out and share the love of Jesus Christ with others. This is the greatest, highest and most important commission that God has given to those of us who have accepted Jesus Christ as our Lord and Savior. Sometimes, depression confines you to your home or your bed, making it really hard for you to get out and about, both mentally and physically. Why would God want that for you?

5) God's greater glory is made manifest when we are healed. God can reveal His glory through illness, but what a testimony we have of His goodness, love and ability to restore us, when we are fully healed by the power of His Spirit!

6) Jesus commands us to heal the sick. As I mentioned earlier, healing is one of the commands that God gives us as part of the Great Commission. If He wanted some of us to be sick, why would He command us to heal others? It would mean that He is a respecter of persons, but Scripture says that He is no respecter of persons. He wants us all to be well!

In *Healing Chronic Illness: By His Spirit, Through His Resources*, I share other reasons why some of us in North America and other developed nations don't believe in supernatural healing, including the fact that it is relatively uncommon in these places (although thankfully is becoming more common as people step out and choose to believe God and His Word!).

For instance, Christians sometimes don't believe that healing is always God's will because, in the Bible, God allowed Job to be afflicted with disease and Paul with a "thorn in the flesh," –the latter of which some theologians teach is disease. If you study the original Greek texts, however, you'll see that Paul's thorn was actually a messenger of Satan sent to torment him. In any case, Paul and Job are not our models; Jesus and His ministry are. God allowed Satan to afflict Job but we are under a different covenant in this day and age: a covenant in which Jesus died for our sins and sicknesses so that we could be set free.

While much of this book contains other tools that God may use to heal you from depression, including natural medicine, know that the simplest and highest way for you to be healed is through your relationship with God and by believing in the sacrifice of His Son, Jesus Christ. It's yours for the taking. So, if you want to stop here because He has fully convicted and convinced you that you can be healed by faith and your relationship with Him alone, then that's great!

If you feel led to pursue additional help, I encourage you to read the rest of the book, to discover some other amazing resources that will help you to be well, in spirit, soul and body. As I mentioned previously, depression is usually a multifactorial problem, and sometimes, addressing the other causes of depression, like a toxic relationship, environmental illness, or an unhealthy diet, are crucial for recovery. Also, God can do a miracle in your mind and body but if you want to remain healed it's a good idea to follow the natural and spiritual laws that He's created for your wellbeing, and which are intended for you to thrive and be healthy in this world. I discuss these throughout this book.

Whatever you decide to do, know that God has provided abundant resources for you to be fully restored from depression, and I believe that He will highlight to you what you most need, throughout the pages of this book as well as elsewhere. May His Spirit bring revelation, refreshment, hope, healing and life abundant to your spirit, soul and body!

Chapter Four

Find Healing for Your Soul

A common cause of depression is trauma or soul wounds, which are created as a result of harm or perceived harm that has been done to us by others. Soul wounds that occur in childhood because of abuse can be especially pernicious and damaging and have long-standing negative repercussions that permeate every aspect of who we are. Soul wounds can also affect how we perceive God, our ability to receive from Him, and the fullness of the life and calling that He's given us.

Most, if not all of us, have soul wounds. The good news is that God has lots of ways to heal your soul that can include simply spending time with Him or receiving healing through the prayers or ministry of another person. As well, mind-body tools such as brain retraining programs can be tremendously helpful for renewing the mind, which is a crucial component of soul health. Mind renewal involves identifying any harmful or lie-based beliefs, thoughts and behaviors that you've learned to adopt as a result of the soul wounds and trauma, and then replacing those with God's truths. An important aspect of this process involves identifying and renouncing what are called harmful inner vows, bitter root judgments and expectations. Following I share with you more about these concepts and how you can apply them to your life, with God's help!

In addition, healing from soul wounds involves identifying and overcoming a poverty mindset, which I've discovered to be common in most people who battle depression caused by early life trauma. In the following section I'll share more about what it means to have a poverty mindset and how you can overcome that, too, and live in the fullness of the life that God intends for you!

You may find that the following mind-renewal tools will be easier to apply within the context of a guided prayer session, along with the help of a trained healing minister, or mature, Spirit-filled counselor. You can apply them on your own in your prayer time with God, but if you battle symptoms of depression or brain fog, are unmotivated, or simply struggle to connect with God, you may reap greater benefit by doing them with the help of a minister or Spirit-filled friend that you trust.

Overcoming a Poverty Mindset

Many of us who have battled depression have been conditioned to live out of a poverty mindset, which can be a major reason why we don't thrive and prosper: in our emotional and physical health, finances, relationships and other areas of life. A poverty mindset isn't about not having enough of something. Rather, it's about *feeling* like you never have enough, and consequently, being tormented by fears of lack and not being able to survive. It's rooted in a fear that you won't be provided for, or that God's definition of provision is for you to live in a garbage dump, eating your neighbor's leftover rice (or some version thereof!). It's expecting that you'll receive just enough to scrape by or believing that God will bless you only if you do everything right.

If you battle a poverty mindset, you may think that you have to beg, scrimp and pinch pennies to make it in the world because there is never enough. Your motto might be, "I have to take care of me because nobody else will." Yet God is a god of abundance and He wants you to have more than enough, not just enough to barely get by!

Some of you may battle a poverty mindset because you felt rejected or abandoned in some way by your parents or primary caregivers early in life. For instance, perhaps throughout your childhood, you felt that your physical and emotional needs weren't provided for, or that they didn't matter. Maybe you thought that all you deserved were leftovers. Maybe you felt ignored or unimportant, or were even told that you were worthless, or had negative words or curses spoken over you.

If so, I believe that these types of scenarios can bring on a poverty mindset, which is in turn linked to what I call an "orphan spirit." Orphans have been conditioned to expect little from their providers, which for you, might now be God. Your parents may have tried their best to provide for you, but what we perceive as children—whether it reflects reality or not—will affect us throughout our lives until we learn to embrace God's truths instead of the lies that we've been programmed to believe.

All of the following are additional indications of a poverty mindset. How many of these do you relate to?:

A). You feel like you don't have enough, and never will

B). You fear not being provided for

C). You put a ceiling on how much you think that God can or wants to give you

D). You feel like you are in "survival mode" daily

E). You are tight-fisted with your resources because you fear losing what you have. Or, you overspend because you think there will be nothing left for tomorrow, so you decide that there is no point in saving your money.

F). You rush through the day to get things done

G). You covet what others have, because you think that God hasn't provided for all of your needs

H). You believe that you don't deserve good things

I). You don't trust God to provide for all of your needs

J). You continually talk about how you are barely making ends meet, or how bad the economy is. You have a victim mentality and often think that other people's lives are better than yours.

K). You make goals based on the desire for money or the need to survive, rather than God's will or the passions that He's placed in your heart

L). You hoard stuff because you fear that there will be nothing for tomorrow

As I mentioned, a poverty spirit isn't about how much you have, but rather, what you perceive you don't have or fears of not being provided for. You can live in a mansion and still live in fear of lack. Conversely, you can live in a shack and feel rich, if you trust God to meet all of your needs.

It's helpful to know whether you are operating out of a poverty mindset, because it can affect your recovery from depression and your relationship with God. This is because you will tend to entertain faulty beliefs about your self-worth and God's provision for you. You can't be at peace if you wonder day to day whether God will meet all of your needs. What's more, a poverty mindset will keep you locked in patterns of belief and behavior that may hinder you from receiving His blessings, because you will either don't feel like you deserve them, or that He doesn't really want to give good things to you.

One obvious way in which a poverty mindset manifests is as financial problems. If you feel like you're barely making it in life or can't get ahead, no matter what you do, it may be because you believe a lie about God's provision for you and what you have to do to receive that. Maybe you find yourself constantly worrying about whether you'll be able to make ends meet, or you take on jobs that you despise, just to pay the bills, even though the work doesn't align with your heart's desires or God's will for your life. Or, maybe you accept low-paying jobs because you don't think that you are able or deserve (probably subconsciously) to make a good living, or you lack confidence in your ability to do better.

These kinds of beliefs can cloud you from seeing and pursuing God's will for your life because they cause you to make decisions out of fear and what seems like a rational need to earn money and survive, rather than out of who and what God has created you to be. And when you aren't doing the things that He's called you to do, this can leave you feeling dissatisfied, empty and even depressed, because He gave you certain gifts and talents, and put specific desires and dreams in your heart. Essentially, when you aren't true to yourself and to who He has called you to be, you live out of alignment with Him and your heart.

You may find yourself battling a poverty mindset in the area of finances for other reasons. Maybe deep down, you don't believe that you deserve good things, or that God needs for you to be poor so that He can build your character. Or maybe you think you aren't smart enough or worthy enough to do those things that He's called you to do.

To overcome a poverty mentality, I encourage you to ask God to show you four things: 1) How He sees you 2) Who you are in Him 3) Who He is in you, and 4) the Kingdom inheritance that He's given you. Then, ask Him how He wants to bless you. As part of this, you may want to do a search online using terms such as, "Scriptures about my identity in Christ" or "how God sees me" which will usually pull up an excellent list of Bible verses for you to meditate on. Then, ask God to highlight the Scriptures that He wants to use to speak to you personally.

Shortly after I surrendered my life to God, I began to dress more elegantly and spend more money on high-quality clothes. Prior to that, I would feel guilty whenever I purchased a nice dress or new pair of shoes, and I realized that it was because throughout my life, I hadn't believed that

I deserved nice clothes. God told me that He wanted to teach me otherwise. As I started to dress better, it helped me to remember that I was royalty in God's Kingdom: His princess and beloved child, to whom He wanted to give beautiful and costly things.

God may not tell you to go buy new clothes. In fact, He may tell you to stop buying clothes and give some of your money to the poor. Maybe buying clothes fills an emotional void for you and has become a substitute for relationship with Him or others. If so, God may want to teach you how to get that emotional need met through Him. Or, He may simply want you to know that it is more blessed to give than to receive, and that there are spiritual rewards that come from giving to others. Maybe He desires to show you how He will provide for you when you do so.

Do you see how God works to remove a poverty mentality? Following are some additional guidelines for vanquishing a poverty mindset from your life.

First, be generous with your finances, as God leads you. Proverbs 3:8-10 tells us that if we are generous, we will reap financial blessings as a result. It says, "Honor the Lord with your wealth, and with the first fruits of all your crops (income); then your barns will be abundantly filled and your vats will overflow with new wine." This means that whatever you receive from God, in the form of income, gifts or other financial dividends, give Him a portion of that income first, before you do anything else with your money. You can do this by contributing to your local church, a charity organization or other ministry. Give some of your money to the beggar on the corner or to the man who lives under the bridge, or to an international relief fund. Or, sponsor a child in a foreign country.

By doing any of these things, you give not only to the organization or person, but also to God, and by giving to Him first you acknowledge that He is the most important priority in your life and that you trust Him to meet your every need. Matthew 25:40 says "Truly I tell you, whatever you did for one of the least of these brothers and sisters of mine, you did for me."

Believe God for the impossible! He wants to bless you with wealth, because the more that you have to contribute to His Kingdom, the more lives you can influence for His Kingdom. There is nothing noble about being poor. Think about it. If your income increased, how many more children in Africa could you feed? How many more missionaries could you sponsor to spread the gospel? Poverty is not godly!

When you are depressed, it's easy to become self-focused and forget about God's Kingdom and the needs of others, but God says that we will prosper when we obey Him and give to His Kingdom. One of the principles of living abundantly in the Kingdom of God is giving. When we don't do this, we become impoverished spiritually as well as financially.

That said, God doesn't withhold His blessings from you just because you feel that you aren't able to give at times, and neither are His blessings contingent upon your performance. What's more, He doesn't want you to give primarily so that you expect to receive something back in return, but rather, because you love Him and care about the welfare of others. As His Word says, God loves a cheerful giver (1 Cor. 9:7). At the same time, spiritual laws govern the world, and the Bible tells us that we will reap what we sow (1 Cor. 1:12) and God wants you to reap abundantly!

As a simple example of how this works, if you speak harshly to someone, chances are, they will respond by being unkind back to you. If you eat junk food regularly, you may feel poorly or even gain weight. These examples illustrate the law of sowing and reaping in action.

Similarly, when you are generous with your finances, time or talents, you demonstrate that you believe and trust that God owns all the resources in the world and has enough to bless you exceedingly, and His Word confirms this. When you give, you will find that God often gives back to you much more than what you gave out!

Further, although God no longer requires His people to give away 1/10th of their income as He did in the Old Testament, many of God's leaders still advocate tithing, or donating, at least the first 10% of your income to Him, for His Kingdom purposes, and as a sign of gratitude toward Him for all that He's done for you. It also shows that you trust Him to meet all of your needs. Don't be surprised if, when you do this, He opens the floodgates of Heaven for you and pours out such a blessing that you can't contain it (Malachi 3:10).

Once, a good friend of mine needed $1,000 to pay off a debt so that the bank wouldn't take her house away from her. She lives in Costa Rica, and at that time and in that place, $1,000 was a significant sum of money. She called me to ask me for help. At the time, I was quite sick and didn't have much money in savings and was living off of my disability check of $1,100 per month, as well as the earnings from my books, which at the time were just enough to pay my bills.

Yet I thought, "How can I *not* help her? Besides, God will honor me and make sure that my needs are met."

I sent her the money from Colorado via MoneyGram, and after she left a MoneyGram serviced bank in San Jose, a city that has had a number of muggings and robberies in recent years, she boarded a bus in San Jose with the wad of cash.

Shortly thereafter, at one of the bus stops, two armed men boarded the bus and proceeded to rob everyone on it! They held pistols to the passengers' heads and took their cell phones, wallets and backpacks...basically, everything. When they got to her seat, one of the men pointed his gun at her, ready to demand that she hand over all of her belongings to him, but his colleague tapped him and said, "Not her. Leave her alone."

It was incredible. The men had robbed everyone on the bus, *except for her*! And in all likelihood, she had probably been carrying more money than any of the other passengers. This event was a powerful reminder to me of God's power, protection and ability to provide, because I knew that His hand had halted the robbers. My friend was elated, and so was I.

But the story gets even better. About a week after I sent her the money, the manager at the apartment complex where I was residing called me and told me that the staff had done a raffle for someone to win a free month of rent...and guess who won? Yours truly! What was even more extraordinary was the fact that the amount of the prize was exactly the amount that I had sent to my friend to pay off her debt.

God was showing me that He could easily return to me everything that I gave out to others, and then some. In other situations, where I have donated money, prayed for people or helped them out in some other way, God has often multiplied the blessing by giving back to me more than what I gave away. It doesn't always happen immediately, and I don't think there is always a noticeable cause and effect with giving, but in general, I notice a tangible payback from God, perhaps just to show me that He's proud of me, that He owns all the resources, and can provide for all of my needs when I am generous toward others.

When we focus on other people's needs, it also tends to be easier for us to look away from our own problems and all that's wrong with our lives. As the Apostle Paul says in Acts 20:35, "In everything I did, I showed you that by this kind of hard work we must help the weak, remembering the words the Lord Jesus himself said: 'It is more blessed to give than to receive.'"

When you give to others out of a spirit of love, you advance the Kingdom of God and please God because you are doing the same works that Jesus did. It also blesses your spirit and draws you closer to God, as you become more like Him. And what better gift is there any way than to witness the joy or thankfulness in someone's eyes when you demonstrate His love to that person? God gives us a sense of peace and joy when we provide for others, and I have often felt His pleasure when I do so.

Society often tells us the opposite, though. The messages that we receive in the media and elsewhere admonish us to consume, hoard and look out for ourselves, because it's a "dog eat dog" world. The media would have you believe that happiness comes from having a nicer car or home, and by being in relationships where others meet your every need, rather than you contributing to theirs.

Yet people who have truly discovered the secret of happiness know that the greatest and highest joy in life is to live selflessly, doing the same works that Jesus did. Such people know that they don't have to work to get their needs met, because God delights to take care of them when they are about His business. God loves us all and provides for us no matter what, but I believe there is increased favor and provision when we give up our lives for the Kingdom and surrender to His will, plans and purposes for our lives. If we are about His business, He will be about ours.

I also believe that we receive increased blessing and favor when we are faithful stewards of the resources that God has given us. If you continually buy things that you don't need, take advantage of or "mooch" off of others, don't pay your taxes, get into debt, or use God's resources for selfish gain, rather than the Kingdom, you may not be as blessed financially as you could be.

God forgives our mistakes and knows that we need help in every area of our lives—indeed, He doesn't condemn you if you have fallen into debt or lived off of others because you don't know how to receive His provision, but He wants you to trust Him with all that you have. Even if you have just a dollar or two to give away, if you are faithful to use that dollar wisely, and/or give it away when He asks you to do so, He can multiply that dollar so that it becomes a hundred, then two hundred, then a thousand, and so on.

Conversely, when you give away everything that you own, or give when God doesn't tell you to, in order to earn favor with people or because you don't believe that you deserve good things; or because a religious spirit tells you to always put others above yourself, these attitudes can indicate that you're under the influence of a poverty mentality, too. Sometimes, we give all of our stuff away, because deep down, we believe that we aren't worthy of good things or we need the approval of others. Yet God admonishes you to love others as yourself, not *instead* of yourself (Mark 12:31).

If you struggle to trust God, and can't seem to get out of living in "survival mode" or out of a poverty mentality, you may find it useful to do some inner healing prayer with a trusted minister or counselor who can help you to identify poverty-based beliefs that are causing you to learn to expect little from God. He or she can then help you to replace those beliefs with the truth about how God sees you and how He so richly wants to provide for your every need!

Following are some verses that demonstrate how God provides for His people. I encourage you to meditate upon these verses and ask God to reveal their deeper meaning for you personally.

Psalm 34:10 "The young lions suffer want and hunger; but those who seek the LORD lack no good thing."

Matthew 6:31-32 "Therefore do not be anxious, saying, 'What shall we eat?' or 'What shall we drink?' or 'What shall we wear?' For the Gentiles seek after all these things, and your heavenly Father knows that you need them all."

Philippians 4:19 "And my God will supply every need of yours according to his riches in glory in Christ Jesus."

Romans 8:32 "He who did not spare his own Son but gave him up for us all, how will he not also with him graciously give us all things?"

Matthew 7:7 "Ask, and it will be given to you; seek, and you will find; knock, and it will be opened to you."

Matthew 7:11 "If you then, who are evil, know how to give good gifts to your children, how much more will your Father who is in heaven give good things to those who ask him!"

Matthew 21:22 "And whatever you ask in prayer, you will receive, if you have faith."

John 14:13-14 "Whatever you ask in my name, this I will do, that the Father may be glorified in the Son. If you ask me anything in my name, I will do it."

John 15:7 "If you abide in me, and my words abide in you, ask whatever you wish, and it will be done for you."

My favorite verse here is Romans 8:32: "He who did not spare his own Son but gave him up for us all, how will he not also, along with Him, graciously give us all things?"

Just ponder the significance of that for a moment. God sacrificed His only Begotten Son on a cross, allowing Him to die a brutal death so that we could be healed and free, here on earth, as well as in the Hereafter. This is the highest expression of love there is. No greater sacrifice could one human being offer to another! If this is true, and God promises to give us all things, then why do we expect so little from Him?

Maybe you are thinking, *Well, if He wanted to give me so much, then why has He allowed me to suffer for so long with depression?* Or, pick your favorite hardship! Maybe you feel resentful and doubt God's provision for you because you've lived for years in a moldy apartment and have been unable to pay your bills. Maybe your car constantly breaks down, and you never seem to have enough money for a vacation, a night out with friends, or all the fun things that other people you know seem to get to do.

Provision is a state of mind though as much as it is a tangible reality. Consider this: a person in a third-world country who lives in a mud hut and eats nothing but rice daily can feel abundantly provided for by God, while a person who has two cars and a mortgage might complain about having a smaller house than his neighbor, and fear that he is constantly one paycheck short of not being able to make ends meet. Which has a poverty mindset? You guessed it, the one with two cars and a mortgage.

Have you truly believed God will provide for you, or have you simply hoped that He would? Have you believed a lie about your worth and how God wants to provide for you? If so, I encourage you to meditate on the Scripture verses that speak of His provision, until the truths contained within them become more real than the lies that you've been conditioned to believe.

As part of eliminating the poverty mindset, it's really beneficial to ask God to show you how He sees you. We are servants of God but we are also His beloved sons and daughters who have been given a huge Kingdom inheritance, and the keys to His Kingdom. He wants us to prosper in every way: in our health, finances, relationships, and every other area of life.

3 John 2 says, "Beloved, I pray that in every way you may succeed and prosper and be in good health [physically], just as [I know] your soul prospers [spiritually]."

I encourage you to meditate on the following verses that relate to your identity in Him, how He sees you, and the inheritance that He's given to you as part of His Kingdom. Following are a few examples. According to His Word, you are:

1. His beloved child —John 1:12
2. The apple of His eye – Psalm 17:8
3. His pearl of great price   Matthew 13:46
4. Precious and honored in His sight – Isaiah 43:4
5. The bride of Jesus Christ— Revelation 19:7
6. The recipient of all His promises – 2 Peter 1:4
7. A co-heir with Jesus — Galatians 4:7
8. The light of the world — Matthew 5:14
9. The righteousness of God in Christ — 2 Corinthians 5:21
10. Forgiven and cleansed of all unrighteousness. – 1 John 1:9

You are not your past, your behavior or whatever has happened to you. You are not a depressed or sick person. You may battle depression, but according to God's Word, you are a new creation, made perfect in Christ, and He loves, cherishes and adores you! The more you allow the truths contained within the Scriptures that I just mentioned to go deep into your DNA and transform you, the less you will find yourself a prisoner of depression, as the "real you" begins to emerge and take center stage in your life. But don't just read the verses; meditate and chew on them, even "do" them! Ask

God to show you what they mean for you personally, and how you can live out the truths contained within them.

Deeply ingrained habits can be hard to break, so you may want to ask God to nudge you whenever you have a thought that is poverty-based, or which doesn't align with His truths and what He says about you. Then, ask Him to give you a word to replace whatever lie the enemy is trying to plant within you at that moment.

On that note, another crucial step for breaking a poverty mentality is to avoid speaking word curses over yourself and others. For instance, if you periodically say things like, "The economy is terrible. I can't afford this. I can't work. Everything is expensive. I have no money. I'm too (fill in the blank) to be able to make it in this world," among other phrases of the like, you will end up creating a self-fulfilling prophecy in your life and feeding the poverty mindset, as you affirm your trust in yourself and circumstances, not God, to provide for you.

We all curse ourselves at times, purposely or inadvertently, so don't be hard on yourself if you realize that you have been speaking lies over yourself. We all battle fear of not being provided for at times, and when things seem scarce, or depression weighs heavily upon you and distorts reality, it's really easy to fall into the trap of worry and unbelief. It may be true that you aren't able to pay all of your bills right now, but I encourage you to say, in the midst of the battle, when it is most difficult to stand on the truth: "God will provide. God will make a way!"

Affirm your belief in Him and choose to trust Him for provision, even if you don't feel like it. We exhibit faith and trust when we publicly proclaim what God says about our situations, regardless of how we feel or how things seem. In the meantime, honor God with your resources by asking Him to help you not waste them, nor overspend, so that you can use what you have wisely.

Another key to removing a poverty mindset and which will help you to cultivate a joyful spirit is to give God thanks for what you have, while resisting the urge to covet what others have. 1 Thessalonians 5:18 says, "In everything give thanks; for this is God's will for you in Christ Jesus." This positions you to receive more from God, and can help to mitigate depression, since giving thanks reminds you of all the great things that God has already done for you.

At the same time, don't seek security in what you own, but only in God. God has a lot to say in His Word about not trusting in riches, which any of us could lose in an instant. For instance, 1 Timothy 6:17 says, "Command those who are rich in this present world not to be arrogant nor to put their hope in wealth, which is so uncertain, but to put their hope in God, who richly provides us with everything for our enjoyment." Let your hope be in God, not in your abilities or what you have.

So, depend on God, not other people, for all of your needs! When we hurt and worry about our ability to provide for ourselves, we tend to look to others to meet our needs. It's human nature. While God uses other people to bless and help us, there is no single person out there who can meet all of your needs. If, through your worst battles with depression, you've felt like nobody has been there for you, I encourage you to remember that Jesus' disciples abandoned Him in his darkest hour at the Garden of Gethsemane. Yet God the Father was with Him to strengthen, sustain and uphold Him. Similarly, God is always with us to do the same for us.

Finally, if you think that you've been entertaining any poverty-based thoughts, I encourage you to ask God for forgiveness, repent for those thoughts and renounce them, and say good-bye to them forever, as you affirm daily His goodness, willingness and ability to meet all of your needs. Philippians 4:19 says, "And my God will meet all your needs according to the riches of his glory in Christ Jesus." (NIV). Choose to believe this truth, despite how you may feel, and you will see it come to fruition!

The Power of Forgiveness and Renouncing Inner Vows, Bitter Root Judgments and Expectations

Note: The following information is based partly upon what I have learned from ministers John Loren and Mark Sandford, authors of the book, *Deliverance and Inner Healing*. John Loren and his wife, Paula Sandford, founded Elijah House, a worldwide inner healing ministry, the mission of which is "to restore the hearts of the fathers to their children, and the hearts of the children to their fathers" (Malachi 4:5-6). The Sandfords ministered inner healing and deliverance for over 40 years, and I have found their teachings and insights invaluable for identifying and

resolving soul wounds, in myself and other people that I
have ministered to. To learn more about their ministry and
to find an Elijah house prayer minister from which you can
get help for your own healing journey, visit: elijahhouse.org.

Identifying and Renouncing Inner Vows

In *Deliverance and Inner Healing*, John Loren and
Mark describe what are called "inner vows," which the
authors define (paraphrased) as harmful determinations or
resolute decisions that we all make, usually as young
children, to protect ourselves.[vii] Inner vows are created as a
result of wounding, trauma, and unmet needs, as well as
expectations about how we believe that life will go for us.

For example, a girl who is raised in an unhappy
household where children are treated as a burden may
subconsciously vow, "I will never have children because they
are a burden and a hindrance to a happy life." When she
becomes an adult, she decides not to have a family, but may
be unaware of the true reason why she doesn't want
children.

Inner vows can lead to depression because rather than
protecting you, they will actually create undesirable
circumstances, such as isolation, and keep you bound in a
prison of your own making, so that you don't enjoy life. They
keep you rooted in bad situations and bad relationships
because of what you believe, even if your heart profoundly
desires to live differently.

We all make inner vows, but we aren't usually aware of
them because most reside in our subconscious. Some vows

are big, while others are small. For instance, if, when you were a child, you were teased because you stuttered when you spoke before your classmates, you may have made an inner vow to never speak in public.

Now, because of that vow, you break out in a sweat and get anxious every time you find yourself accidentally standing before an audience to speak. Because of this, you miss out on opportunities that God has for you as a speaker or a public figure, because you don't want to speak before groups of people.

Another common, and deeper inner vow that some people (especially women) make as a result of early childhood abuse by their fathers is, "I will never trust or be vulnerable with a man." If you were severely molested, you may make a stronger vow, such as "I will never let a man take advantage of me again."

Or, perhaps you were raised in a household where you were criticized every time you gave an opinion about something, so you made inner vows to not feel or express your opinions with others. I made such vows and as a child, for years, I hardly spoke to anyone at school. Teachers thought that I had a learning disability because I wouldn't respond when they addressed me, and kids made fun of me, "the mute."

Then one day, years later, God made a promise to me: "The voice that was silenced will one day be a voice for thousands." What an amazing promise that was! And I am seeing that promise come to fruition now, as I have published books that have reached thousands of people and have had the opportunity to share God's love publicly; on the radio, through podcasts, social media and webinars, in churches and elsewhere.

Paradoxically though, inner vows create the opposite effect of what you intend and, instead of protecting you, they often bring about the *exact* situation that you are trying to avoid! In *Deliverance and Inner Healing,* the authors cite several examples of this, including a woman who vowed that she would never date an abusive alcoholic because her dad had been an alcoholic. Yet she ended up marrying one, multiple times! At the time that she had married these men, they weren't drinkers, but all become alcoholics at some point during her marriage to them—and she ended up suffering the same consequences of abuse in her marriage as in her childhood.

In order to get set free from this harmful pattern, the woman had to repent of her inner vow to not marry an alcoholic, and forgive her father and former husbands, as she also repented for and renounced any judgments that she held against them. This broke the chain of dysfunctional marriages in her life.

This woman's experience occurred because of what's called the law of sowing and reaping, which is described in Galatians 6:7-9. Here, it says, "Do not be deceived, God is not mocked [He will not allow Himself to be ridiculed, nor treated with contempt nor allow His precepts to be scornfully set aside]; for whatever a man sows, this and this only is what he will reap. For the one who sows to his flesh [his sinful capacity, his worldliness, his disgraceful impulses] will reap from the flesh ruin and destruction, but the one who sows to the Spirit will from the Spirit reap eternal life."

What we reap in life is based largely upon our judgments and beliefs about others, God, and ourselves. And, it is a spiritual principle that when we judge others and attempt to protect ourselves through those judgments, we will actually do greater harm to ourselves. We can make the very situations that we are trying to protect ourselves from to come to fruition!

We all have inner vows, and I don't think that God requires you to figure out and renounce every single one, but you may want to ask Him if there are any major core vows that are contributing to your lack of wellbeing and which are hindering you from being able to move forward in life. When He reveals them to you, simply repent for and sincerely renounce them before Him, as you also forgive those who may have triggered you to make them in the first place. Then, affirm your trust in Him to protect you from whatever it is that you made a vow for or against, and ask Him to help you to replace any harmful beliefs associated with those vows with His truths.

Again, don't think that you have to figure it all out! I think that some of us can have a love encounter with God that will wash away all of the fear, bitterness, unforgiveness and resentments that we have buried in our soul, and I don't think that renouncing inner vows is a requirement for healing. God deals with us all differently, but He may decide that this is one way in which He wants to heal you. So ask

Him, and see what He has to say. Remember, this is all for your own good, because inner vows can contribute to depression, and He wants to set you free!

Renouncing Bitter Root Judgments and Expectations

Inner vows go hand-in-hand with what are called "bitter root judgments and expectations." A bitter root judgment is a negative judgment or expectation about how circumstances will go for you in life. For instance, if your mother abandoned you in childhood, you may develop the belief, or bitter root judgment, that women aren't trustworthy, and consequently, begin to expect that all of your friends, or your spouse (if you are a man) will leave you. Like inner vows, most bitter root judgments and expectations are created in childhood.

The flawed lens through which we view others then causes us to judge them, God, and ourselves wrongly. We all have many judgments in our soul, which is why we need to learn to live out of our spirit, which, in cooperation with the Holy Spirit, teaches us how to judge rightly.

Judgments can also keep us from being healed, because as long as we have judgments about ourselves, God and others, it means that we haven't truly forgiven those who were the cause or initial trigger for us to develop those judgments in the first place. So, if you think that you've forgiven someone, but you still negatively judge their behavior, then it means that you are probably still harboring bitterness and unforgiveness in your heart against them.

Bitter root judgments and expectations can cause us to end up making such serious mistakes as marrying the wrong person or getting into abusive relationships with people whose behavior will end up reflecting that of the person(s) we are judging. According to John Sandford, we might marry someone that is, or who "becomes" the parent we judged, only worse! [viii] The example of the woman who married two alcoholics is one example of this.

Bitter root judgments and expectations are ultimately the result of unforgiveness, so I encourage you to first ask God whom you may still need to forgive; in your past, present or future. That person may be you or even Him. Along with that, ask Him what judgments you are holding against those people and what you have learned to expect in life and from others because of those judgments. James 5:16 says, "Therefore confess your sins to each other and pray for each other so that you may be healed. The prayer of a righteous person is powerful and effective."

When I did this myself, with the help of the Holy Spirit, I realized that I was operating out of a whole lie-based system of beliefs and behaviors, but there were a few judgments that were key to the bondage and depression that I was in. So rather than deal with every lie and bitter root judgment since the time of my birth, Holy Spirit had me focus on those that were at the root of my problems and most significantly impacting my life negatively.

I repented for the judgments, along with any inner vows that were attached to those, and then released and forgave the people in my life who had been the triggers for creating those inner vows, judgments and expectations, as I also forgave myself for operating out of a faulty belief system. The bitter thoughts still came up from time to time after that, but by continually bringing them to Jesus and renouncing them and choosing His thoughts over those of my unsanctified soul, over time, I became increasingly freed from their effects.

One unfortunate consequence of bitter root judgments and expectations is that they can program your behavior and beliefs so that you remain locked in dysfunctional living patterns for years. Breaking lifelong beliefs and thought patterns isn't easy because they have become your modus operandi, or habitual way of being, and they deeply influence the way you live. Your decisions, no matter how well intentioned, can be guided by them until God removes them, which is why you need Him to show you where and how you are judging others, yourself or Him. He can then teach you His life-giving truths, and how to live and walk in those truths.

Bitter root judgments and expectations encourage depression when they are pervasive because they keep you locked in dysfunctional, life-draining living patterns. And, it's difficult to be happy if you're walking around angry and judging others all the time because of past wounds!

We all want to make good decisions, but the truth is, until your soul is healed, you will tend to make decisions based on your wounding as well as upon God's will, if you are seeking Him. However, the more you focus on strengthening your spirit and your relationship with God, the more your soul will also be healed as a byproduct of knowing Him, but part of this involves you making the choice to discard old, unhealthy beliefs and renew your mind daily with His truths.

Ephesians 4:21-24 says, "If in fact you have [really] heard Him and have been taught by Him, just as truth is in Jesus [revealed in His life and personified in Him], that, regarding your previous way of life, you put off your old self [completely discard your former nature], which is being corrupted through deceitful desires, and be continually renewed in the spirit of your mind [having a fresh, untarnished mental and spiritual attitude], and put on the new self [the regenerated and renewed nature], created in God's image, [godlike] in the righteousness and holiness of the truth [living in a way that expresses to God your gratitude for your salvation]."

Even if God supernaturally heals you from depression, you'll still need to practice mind renewal as described in Ephesians 4:21-24, repent for any unforgiveness and bitter root judgments that you have toward others, and daily put His truths into practice, or the depression may return. This is because most often, depression isn't just a physical or chemical problem, but an emotional and spiritual one, too.

Sanctification is part of the healing process, yet just as supernatural as receiving a healing miracle in your body, because it is God who enables you to forgive others and renew your mind, and it is He who ultimately heals your emotions. The good news is, as He helps you to choose His thoughts daily, you will find that your mind, emotions, and body will, over time, become permanently re-wired and aligned with His truths.

If this sounds challenging, that's because it can be. Yet if you have accepted Jesus Christ as your Lord and Savior, and received the Holy Spirit, you now have the ability to believe, think and walk as Jesus Christ—even if at times, it doesn't seem like it! You have His mind but aligning your mind with His is still a process (1 Cor. 2:16). Still, know that you are fully equipped to do this, in cooperation with His Spirit, because, as He says, "He has given us all that we need for life and godliness" (2 Peter, 1-3, paraphrased).

Once you have the Author of all life living inside of you, you are no longer a slave to soul wounds, lies, or the programming of your mind. But again, walking in the fullness of that is a process, and receiving the full revelation of what He's given you by His Spirit can take time.

I know this sounds challenging when you are swimming in the depths of depression. I know it can seem like your thoughts, decisions and destiny are based on your flawed or broken DNA, but remember, as a child of God, you technically now have God DNA. If you aren't experiencing the reality of that, it's probably because it hasn't become a full heart revelation to you yet. But don't despair! Ask God to reveal and impart to you the revelation of the fullness of who you are in Him, who He is in you, and the power that He has given you to overcome. You can't just "get it" by willpower. He must show you. The revelation has to go past your intellect, into your heart. Intellectual agreement does not produce change, only a heart revelation can.

If you yet feel powerless to think God's thoughts, because you believe that your chemistry is just too messed-up, or you have just endured too much trauma in your life, I encourage you to meditate upon the fact that "with God, all things are possible" (Matthew 19:26). Over and over again! You can't do it on your own, anyway, messed up chemistry or not. You never could. Even if you didn't battle depression, it is impossible to live a Spirit-filled life without the help of God because the changes that He makes in you aren't at the level of your human flesh, but your spirit. How much more do you need to rely upon Him and trust Him, when you are battling a condition that has greatly affected your thoughts and emotions, and even your body?

In any case, your mind is very powerful, and if you need further evidence for this, consider reading the books of neuroscience researchers Norman Doidge, MD, author of *The Brain's Way of Healing: Remarkable Discoveries and Recoveries from the Frontiers of Neuroplasticity* and *The Brain That Changes Itself: Stories of Personal Triumph from the Frontiers of Brain Science* and Annie Hopper's *Wired for Healing*. These may help to convince you that your brain and the rest of your body *can* heal based on what you think and say!

In the meantime, as you are led, consider doing the following step-by-step prayer to remove bitter root judgments, expectations and inner vows from your life. This may take some time, so don't rush the process.

1) First, ask God what core bitter root judgments, expectations and inner vows you have made in your life; about yourself, God and others, that may be hindering your healing. Write them down. Ask Him to reveal the lies that you have believed about Him, yourself and others.

2) Confess these, and then repent for entertaining them, one by one. Then renounce them, one by one. Ask God to show you instances in your life when those judgments and vows have played a role in your words, circumstances and decision-making, and the adverse consequences that you've suffered as a result. Then, ask Him to replace every vow with His truths and expectations for your life, and to remind you of these truths when the old thoughts try to rise up again—which they most often will.

Again, I recommend writing down what He shares with you during this time, so that you have a list of His truths at the ready, to refer to whenever the lies try to re-emerge. Over time, His truths will become wired into your brain chemistry, rather than the lie-based beliefs.

3) As part of your confession, forgive those people in your life who were the triggers for you adopting the lie-based beliefs and thought patterns. For example, you might say, "Lord, I forgive my dad, and I ask you to forgive me for judging him for his anger, lack of kindness

and inattention toward me. Forgive me for resenting him and carrying forth those same attitudes and traits into my present relationships, and for expecting the same treatment from other men."

Because sinful thoughts can be deeply ingrained, you'll want to ask God to help you to become aware of them whenever they rise up and you are tempted to "buy into" them. Mind renewal can be challenging, but sometimes using tools like the brain training programs that I mentioned in Chapter Two can help to provide a framework for mind renewal that makes the process much easier.

One sample prayer that you could pray as part of this process is as follows: "In the Name of Jesus, I renounce the bitter root expectation that (insert the lie-based thought here) and the sinful behaviors that it has caused in my life, and I declare them to be dead on the Cross of Jesus Christ. Lord, please bring this behavior or belief to death by the power of Your Cross. Remove my old, unhealthy thought patterns and replace them with your truths. Give me a new heart and new eyes that I may see my loved ones and others the way that you see them. Thank you, in the name of Jehovah Rapha, or Jesus Christ, my healer."

Forgiveness: A Cornerstone to Recovery

You may already know by now that a major key to freedom from depression is forgiveness. It has often been said that when you forgive others, you will set a prisoner free, and that prisoner is yourself. So forgive, not only because Jesus tells you to do so, but also so that you may be healed and made whole.

If you don't feel like forgiving, just know that forgiveness isn't about having fuzzy feelings toward the people who have offended or hurt you. Rather, it is simply about surrendering to Jesus your right to hold a judgment against them. It does not justify their sins nor remove their accountability for those sins, and neither does it mean that you should remain in relationship with them.

When you forgive the people in your past and present that have offended you, you allow God to be the judge and jury over them. This frees you from the burden of having to be the judge and bring your offenders to justice! This is great news, because it means that you don't have to carry the burden for their wrongdoing. God will requite you and recompense you for the damage that was done to you because of their sin or offenses against you. He says, "Vengeance is mine; I will repay" (Romans 12:19).

You don't have to worry. He'll make it up to you in the end, and He is a fair, honest judge in whom you can trust. If you have difficulty forgiving others, a great book on forgiveness that I highly recommend is TD Jakes' *Let It Go*.

God wants you to forgive those who have hurt you for another reason. All of us are sinful, and God tells us that if we don't forgive others, He won't forgive us for our sins. Matthew 6:14-15 says, "For if you forgive men when they sin against you, your heavenly Father will also forgive you. But if you do not forgive men their sins, your Father will not forgive your sins."

This is a pretty serious statement! Consider this: in the eyes of God, all of us have crucified Jesus. We have all betrayed Him, spat on Him, and despised Him. We have all been the people who mocked Him as He died on a cross, and because of this, none of us deserves His love or to live forever with Him in Eternity. Yet, He gave up the life of His only Begotten Son for us, so that we could be forgiven and restored to a perfect relationship with Him. If He did that, then the least we can do is forgive those who have hurt us, as He has forgiven us for rejecting Him and murdering His Son Jesus.

If you are saying to yourself, "I wouldn't have rejected Jesus," consider this: We have all rejected Him by our thoughts and actions at times. We have despised Him by not acknowledging Him or His sacrifice, by not believing His promises or His Word, by not accepting His love, by not loving others or ourselves, and by not living in obedience to Him. All of us are guilty of doing these things. We need forgiveness and much as those who have hurt us need to be forgiven. We all need God's mercy and grace. Anyway, we all have our perspectives about things that have happened in the past, and we don't know what pains those who have hurt us might be carrying, too, which caused them to sin against us.

If you've been greatly hurt by the people in your life, it can be difficult to let go of bitterness and resentment. It may take time for you to fully release them from your judgments and anger, but remember, with God, all things are possible! Only He can change your emotions, but it is up to you to decide whether you want to forgive. If, in your heart, you decide to do so, you may still feel anger towards the person(s) that you are forgiving, but over time, and as you repeatedly affirm your decision to forgive, if your decision is sincere, God will take that decision and change your emotions. It may be like peeling an onion, and you may need to acknowledge multiple times that you forgive the person(s) who have hurt you, especially if the anger or hurt repeatedly rises up within you. Yet if your sincere desire is to see the person(s) through God's eyes and love them as He does, He will certainly help you to do that.

I have found that when I don't want to forgive, it's because I am entertaining a spirit of entitlement that says, "I'm not as bad as this person. I would never do to them what they did to me." Our tendency is to think that we are better than those who have harmed us, and that we are incapable of hurting them in the same the way that they have hurt us. But to God, all sin is the same and leads to the same judgment or end, which is an eternity without Him. He admonishes us to forgive for our sake though, because anger, bitterness, rage, resentment and other negative emotions keep us bound in depression, as well as separated from God on some level. They also make us sick, as many scientific studies have shown, and keep us in a prison of our own making.

When those of us who have accepted Jesus Christ as our Lord and Savior feel a sense of entitlement or have judgments against loved ones or others who have hurt us, it is as if we take lightly or forget about the priceless gift of Jesus' sacrifice for us. We forget about His blood that was shed upon the Cross, and His body that was mercilessly broken so that we could be fully forgiven, set free and reconciled to God for Eternity. He died a brutal death for us; the least we can do in exchange is forgive those who have offended us.

Anyway, consider this: your anger never hurts the one who hurt you, only you! Again, sometimes the pain that others have caused us is so great that we feel like we can't forgive and release that anger, no matter how hard we try.

God only wants your decision so that He can change your emotions, but the decision must come from the heart. It can't be a flippant, "Well, I suppose I'll forgive him..." or a half-hearted choice, or you may remain in bondage. Still, you may have to forgive the person many times before your emotions change, but that's OK. God will take your decision and change your heart, either instantaneously or over time.

If there are people in your life, including yourself and/or God, that you have wanted to truly forgive, but found yourself battling ongoing thoughts of bitterness, even for years, ask God what it is that you need to know; what is hidden in your heart, and what lie you may be believing, that is causing the bitterness to remain. Do this, so that you can be released once and for all from that pain and rage! Ask Him to help you to do what you cannot do in your flesh. Ask Him to give you His perspective on those people (even if it's you!) who have hurt you, and to help you see them as He does.

Matthew 18:21-22 says, "Then Peter came to Him and asked, 'Lord, how many times will my brother sin against me and I forgive him and let it go? Up to seven times?' Jesus answered him, 'I say to you, not up to seven times, but seventy times seven.'" Forgive, and keep on forgiving!

Chapter Five

Overcome Your Life's Losses

Loss is a major and important cause of depression. When it's a one-time event that causes the loss, like the passing on of a loved one or a job loss, the grief or depression that it causes can be intense, but for many, it tends to resolve more easily than great losses that are ongoing, especially those that originate in childhood.

The depression I battled due to Lyme disease and childhood trauma was exacerbated by many losses that I had suffered because of the disease. I spent most of my 30s and early 40s largely housebound, too sick at times to get out and about and do much beyond making runs to the grocery store, pharmacy, or my doctor.

The isolation was crippling. I lived alone during the majority of time that I was severely ill and the lack of face-to-face interaction with people, coupled with an inability to do things, meant that I spent many hours fighting hopelessness. When I called friends, they were kind and tried to be sympathetic to my challenges, but they didn't understand my battle and didn't know how to relate to me, nor I to them. I was envious of their lives and they were tired of hearing about mine, because I felt I didn't have much to talk about except my struggles.

In the meantime, I observed as they did fun things such as go on trips to the mountains or to conferences, picnics, classes, dinners and get-togethers. I watched as friends my age got married, had families, became involved in ministry, established their careers, traveled, bought houses, and did all those things that healthy people in their 30s often do. It was like everyone around me was moving forward, involved in life, while for a long time, every year of my existence looked the same.

For a long time, the routine didn't change much, either. I would get up at 10 or 11 AM and spend the first two hours of my day just trying to coerce my body and brain to get going. Then, I would attempt to pray and spend time with God. I say, "attempt" because some days, I was too brain-fogged or exhausted to pray, and on those days, I would just listen to some worship music or lie in bed, soaking in His presence.

I would spend the rest of my day doing medical research and treatments and using what little physical and mental energy that I had to write. I socialized, traveled and attended events whenever I could, but often, social events were a painful reminder of the life that I was missing out on and I couldn't usually get out often or for long.

I share this to give you an example of some of the losses that I've faced in my life that made my battle with depression more difficult, and to let you know that there is healing from the grief caused by those losses. I know because God has started to redeem much what I've lost. While I still battle regret at times, He continually reminds me of the amazing, wonderful things that He's doing in my life now and how there is redemption and restoration for every trial that I've faced, here as well as in the Hereafter.

For instance, because of what I have suffered, I have had the opportunity to author or co-author 14 wellness books; to minister with great anointing, empathy, wisdom and compassion to others who are sick, and to meet and now spend my life with the most loving man that I've ever known! God has redeemed my trials in other ways; perhaps most importantly, by using them to teach me how to live a healthier, more godly lifestyle.

If you've faced serious losses of any kind, and you haven't processed the grief that inevitably results from those losses, chances are, the depression that you battle is at least partly related to those losses. Loss can make you bitter and angry: perhaps at God, yourself and even others. You may even blame those whom you perceived to be the cause of your losses, unless, of course, you forgive them, which is a crucial component of healing from loss.

The sad, inevitable truth is that we can't ever get back the years that we've lost to bad relationships, a poor upbringing, a difficult disease, a draining job, addictions or unhealthy lifestyle choices. One of the most painful things about life is that we only have so many years on this earth, and when many of those years seem to be squandered on sickness, fruitless endeavors and unhealthy relationships, after a while, the grief and regret over what we perceived we've lost can lead us to despair. Even worse is when you feel like your life continues to be wasted because depression seems to throw a dark cloud over everything that you do; indeed, over your very existence, and you can't see a way out.

Your losses may be similar to mine, or they may be different. Maybe you are fighting depression after the loss of a long-term relationship or marriage that didn't work out. Maybe you've lost a child, parent or spouse, and just can't seem to resolve the grief, even after many years. Maybe you've had to say good-bye to a job that you loved. Maybe the depression you battle is due to an abusive relationship in the present, or an abusive upbringing in the past. Or maybe you were abandoned or never felt loved as a child by your primary caregivers or by God, and those emotions have carried over into your relationship with God today. Maybe He seems just as distant or as unkind as your mother, father or other caregiver.

I've observed that the most refractory and difficult type of depression to overcome, for most people, is that which is due to childhood trauma. This may be because abuse in childhood tears at the very fabric of a person's identity, because children look to their parents for affirmation and get their identity initially from their parents or primary caregivers. So, if your caregivers were critical toward you, or communicated or behaved in a way that caused you to feel like a nuisance, worthless or defective, then chances are, you battle lie-based beliefs about your value, worth and identity—which can create a setup for a lifetime of misery. Unless of course, you have met God and experienced His amazing love for you.

Unraveling the harmful beliefs and lie-based thinking that is created by lack of proper caregiving can be a challenge, but when you truly know God, then it makes things a whole lot easier, if not always easy. But you can rejoice, because God is actually the perfect father and mother and caregiver, and His love can heal you and make up for any deficits from your childhood. Nothing is too hard for Him! Most of our parents tried their best, but even the most loving and godly of parents fall short of His perfection.

In addition to forgiving those who have hurt you, I urge you to not continually look to the past and mull over and regret the things that you've lost. This will reinforce negative pathways in your brain, instead of helping you to create new, healthier ones! Instead, meditate upon how God wants to bless your life in the present. I once read somewhere that we spend most of our time regretting the past and fearing the future, and in so doing, miss out on the present.

You may only have two years of life ahead of you, or you may have twenty, or forty. None of us knows how many days we'll be here on earth, so all we can do is live the best lives we can, where we are at right now. If you're older and feel like your entire life has been a waste because, for example, you had a terrible upbringing and were married to an abusive spouse for 40 years, you may struggle even more now to believe that your life hasn't been in vain. You may also feel this way if up until now, you haven't been in relationship with God or haven't served Him as you've wanted to.

If so, know that you can have a new beginning—starting today! It doesn't matter how old you are, because your life doesn't end when you leave this world. In fact, it will only be beginning, as you'll continue to have plenty of opportunities to be in rewarding relationships and to serve God, here as well as in the Hereafter. Death is only a doorway into another realm of fulfilling relationships, work and intimacy with God. You have important assignments in Heaven, as well as here on earth! So, make the most of today, knowing that today is the beginning of the rest of your life, which will last forever.

When you're tempted to recall the problems or losses from your past, and look at what's behind you, or compare your life to that of someone who seems to have it better than you, make a mental note or write down all of the blessings that God has given you now, and affirm those aloud, rather than allowing your mind to ruminate.

Another tool for overcoming loss is to make a decision daily to live for Eternity, and be in this world, but not of it (John 17:14–19). In my worst moments, I've found that while it's important to follow the calling that God has placed upon my life—and I have greater joy when I do—when I can detach myself from the things of this world, and let go of all of the expectations that I have for my life, I have more peace. God encourages us to be in the world but not of it, because earth isn't our home: Heaven is. Second Corinthians 5-6 states that when we are at home in our physical bodies and in this world, we are away from God. That's a difficult reality for some of us in America to accept and understand, since most of us have lived in relative comfort and opportunity compared to most of the world and may not really mind chasing after a "creature comfort" existence. At least, it seems like a better option for some of us than spending Eternity in a realm that we know very little about!

The church has even communicated the message at times that a prosperous life in Jesus means having riches, glowing health and perfect relationships. While it *can* mean these things, I believe that prosperity in Jesus Christ is more like what the Apostle Paul said while in prison: "In any and every circumstance I have learned the secret [of facing life], whether well-fed or going hungry, whether having an abundance or being in need" (Philippians 4:12). (Note: Some Bible translations say, "I have learned the secret of contentment" here).

The world seems to communicate to us that happiness and peace come from having everything that we want; from riches, to the right man (or woman), to the right house. To some extent, financial prosperity and comfort can bring us temporary, fleeting happiness, but higher joy and lasting peace come from letting go of our need for things to go a certain way, for circumstances to be perfect, and for our every whim to be fulfilled. God cares about our needs and has even put certain desires in our heart, but He wants to meet them in His way and in His timing.

When you lay your plans, hopes and desires at His feet, you can be at peace knowing that He will help cause those things to come to pass in your life, if those desires are part of His plan for your life. He also wants you to live for His eternal purposes, not temporary comforts or pleasures. Incidentally, this will bring you greater peace than if you were to pursue peace through the same avenues as the world.

When I first learned about the Christian concept of "dying to self and living for Christ" I immediately pictured a God who was asking me to deny my personality, needs and identity. What I didn't understand until I got to know Him a little was that He cared about my needs, but that He wanted to meet them in His way, not mine, since He, being my Heavenly Father, knew what I needed much better than I did. As His word says: "And my God will liberally supply (fill until full) your every need according to His riches in glory in Christ Jesus" (Philippians 4:19).

Dying to yourself means surrendering to His will and purposes for your life, and obeying Him daily, knowing that this, in the end, will bring you greater peace and joy than if you tried to acquire for yourself all of the things that you think you need for a life of blessing and abundance. Don't try to collect blessings for yourself, but rather, let Him bless you! Dare to trust Him to provide all that you need: financially, relationally, in your health and all other areas of your life.

Another antidote to depression that's caused by past or present loss is to intentionally thank God daily for the things that He's given you now. That could mean expressing gratitude for something as simple as the beautiful comforter on your bed, the nice view that you have of your neighbor's garden from your office window, your morning coffee, or the good night's sleep that you got last night. It also means being thankful for the more important things, like the relationships that God has put into your life—even the difficult ones, which teach you patience and perseverance, and the ability to love everyone—your relationship with Him, and the lessons that He's teaching you daily. We can all find things to be thankful for, if we just look.

Being thankful is one of those things that you've probably heard that you should do or which you've been told to do dozens of times, yet isn't it interesting how the simplest of instructions that God gives us, such as being thankful for all things, are the most powerful and yet most easily forgotten?

Perhaps it's because His mandate to be thankful seems too easy, or we don't know how powerfully it can change us, so we don't do it. Or maybe we don't feel grateful toward Him because we hurt so much, so remembering or desiring to do it daily is a challenge.

I encourage you though to take five or ten minutes daily to thank God for all that He's given you, because in the spiritual realm, this positions you to receive even greater blessings, since one way that blessings are released is through gratitude. Cultivating gratitude also helps you to find and appreciate the good in your life today, rather than regretting all of the things that you've lost in life up until now and can help to shift your mood and focus in a more positive direction.

It's also important to thank God simply because He is worthy of your honor and praise! He has given all of us the gift of eternal life through Jesus Christ, and that should be enough for us to want to bow down on our face forever and thank Him for His goodness, mercies, grace and loving kindness toward us. We aren't entitled to His love or to live with Him in Eternity; all of us have sinned or fallen short of His glory. So the fact that God would give His only Begotten Son as a living sacrifice for our sake, just so that we could be with Him forever, ought to be enough to convince us to cultivate an attitude of gratitude toward Him. (Notice this is the one place where I will put a "should" and an "ought"!)

Finally, if you've never fully processed and released the emotions resulting from the major losses that you've experienced in life, I encourage you to ask God to help you to do that. You may want to work with a trusted minister or counselor, especially if you know that you've endured great losses but have not been able to access and release the powerful emotions that are created by those, and which may even be buried deep in your psyche.

Know this, though—it's not godly to stuff your emotions. As I mentioned earlier, this can make you sick and/or perpetuate the depression. Ironically, when you release all of the anger, rage, and sadness that has accumulated from your life's losses, God can then more easily come in and heal you from them.

Don't be afraid to be real with Him! I used to meet with a counselor who had such an anointing from God that oil would flow supernaturally from his hands. He held ministry meetings every Friday night, and at those meetings, it wasn't uncommon to see fragments of gold dust, gems and oil appear on his hands and on the floor. The attendees would often get covered in gold dust, too! He is one of the godliest men that I've ever met. He had a lot of authority in the Spirit, and a tremendous love for God.

One day, while I was expressing to him the anger that I felt toward God because of all the horrible things that had happened to me in my life, he reached behind his sofa to hand me a tennis racquet. He then told me to start beating one of the couch pillows that I had been sitting on.

He said, "I want you to tell God how mad you are at Him right now. Go on, let it out!" He then proceeded to cheer me on as He encouraged me to beat the pillow to a pulp, and let out all the accumulated years of anger, rage, grief and disappointment.

At first, when he told me to do this, I thought, *Really? God isn't going to strike me down with a bolt of lightning if I do this?* It was hard to comprehend that I didn't have to sanitize my pain with Him and could yell and curse as much as I wanted to, and He wouldn't get angry with me for it. The minister was encouraging me to let my unedited thoughts and emotions out and had not one condemning word to say after I released a litany of ugly words as I whacked the pillow.

Instead, after my rant, he came up to me and gave me a hug. Then, God spoke through him and said (paraphrased): "My precious daughter: My heart aches for you. I am grieved and so very sorry for all of the terrible tragedies that you have suffered throughout your life, and for the painful darts and arrows that have been inflicted upon you by those who have misrepresented Me and My love to you. They too, were wounded, and didn't realize what they were doing.

"Know that I am your Heavenly Father, and that you are My beautiful princess and daughter, in whom I deeply rejoice and delight! I adore you, I cherish you, and I want the very best for you, and I will restore to you all of the years that the locusts have stolen away. I will heal you, and I will use you to heal multitudes. On behalf of all those who have or will ever hurt you, will you please forgive Me?" (In other words, forgive them).

As tears rolled down my face, I felt the love of God enveloping me in a warm embrace. He wasn't angry for my insolence, lack of faith, or irreverence, because He knew I was hurting—His heart ached for me, and for my restoration. That's love. That's grace. That's mercy!

The release that I experienced that day opened the door for God to come in and heal some of the grief from my past and replace it with His love. It wasn't an overnight process, but since that day with the counselor, I began to feel more empowered and hopeful about my recovery and was able to believe on a deeper level that God truly loved me, just as I was, and even through my pain.

God also used many other people over the years, to speak similar truths into my life. These helped me tremendously, to remain encouraged and hopeful through many years of difficulty and enabled me to keep my eyes on God's promises, purposes and plans for my life.

For instance, I once attended a meeting in which David Wagner, Founder of Father's Heart Ministries, was speaking, and God spoke a word through him to me. He said, "You have a healing ministry from the inside out! You have special authority over cancer, depression, diabetes, bitterness and a poverty spirit!"

Another prophet, Shirley Strand, of New Wind of the Spirit Ministries, once said to me, "Connie, you will be known as the lady who heals Lyme disease! Your ministry is to multitudes and it is for *now*."

These words from God so blessed, uplifted and encouraged me! I received many, many other words, too— and not just from others, but in my quiet time with God. I believe He spoke to me so powerfully because I sought Him so fervently, and because He knew I needed it.

He will speak to you, too! So feel free to be yourself with Him and let Him know how you truly feel. Once you release your pain to Him, ask Him to help you to renounce and repent for any wrong beliefs, attitudes, thoughts or behaviors that you've harbored against yourself, Him and others, just as I described in the previous chapter. Again, repent means to "turn around, or turn away from," so by repenting, you are simply making a commitment to turn away from the ungodly beliefs, thoughts and behaviors that you've held on to, and then let them go.

Then, ask God to fill the void where that pain and all the lies of the enemy once resided, with His hope, encouragement, joy, peace, love and a vision for your future. Chances are, He'll speak words to you that are far more positive, encouraging and hopeful than anything else that you've been thinking up until then. Or, He may give you a vision or a dream, or send someone into your life to help you to believe that you will be healed, and that your future can and will be more prosperous, peaceful and joyful than it is right now.

You may have to do this process a few times, or even many times, until the pain is gone. Regardless, trust that God will meet you where you are at, and help you, no matter what, because He loves you deeply and passionately, and will never, ever give up on you!

Chapter Six

Discover Your Life's Purpose

God lives in you, but you also live in Him (1 John 4:13), and He expresses Himself uniquely through you, according to the character, personality and gifts that He's given you. When you have accepted Jesus as your Lord and Savior, this means that you have the Author of all life living inside of you, and that you have been given the commission, honor and privilege of doing exactly the same works as He did. This includes sharing His love and gift of salvation with others, healing the sick, teaching and instructing others, and loving people in the same way that He did, and still does.

No matter the condition of your soul, you are capable of loving as God loves, if His Spirit lives within you, and your human spirit has been regenerated and is now intimately connected to His. You may not feel qualified or empowered to live as He did, especially if you battle depression on a daily basis, but the more God shows you who you truly are in Him, who He is in you, and the magnificence and magnitude of what He's given you, the more you'll be able to live according to His Spirit, rather than according to how you may feel.

Our spirits soar and thrive when we do the things that God has called and commissioned us to do, even if our soul and body might not agree at first. Often though, when you obey God, your whole being will eventually come into alignment with your spirit, if you sincerely desire to do that which He has created you to do, and you obey wholeheartedly when He gives you the commission.

As I mentioned, I believe that God wants us to share the love of Jesus Christ and the message of His salvation with others, within the larger scope of our unique individual mission in this world. God has designed you with a specific purpose in mind, and He gave you desires, talents, abilities and gifts to fulfill that purpose and mission. Many of us, if we were honest with ourselves though, don't feel like we are walking in the fullness of all that God has called us to be.

I believe this is for many reasons, foremost among these, fear and a lack of knowledge about the abilities that He's given us, our authority in Him, and who He has made us to be. Maybe you feel disqualified to do what He's called you to do, or you don't trust Him to lead, equip and guide you in His plan for your life.

Maybe you fear that God has called you to do something scary or boring with your life, and you believe that if you lose your life and surrender it to Him, it will mean walking into a world of misery where your needs won't be met.

I used to believe that serving God meant that I would become more depressed, because the Bible indicates that we will share in His sufferings when we serve Him (Philippians 3:10 and Romans 8:17). While some types of suffering, like illness or trauma, can foster depression, I don't believe this is the kind of suffering He calls us to. As I have come to know Him, I now believe that when we are truly serving Him, we will find joy and peace through the kind of suffering that He allows us to endure, which is usually some form of persecution for loving Him and sharing His message of salvation with others (Matthew 5:10). But those who are called to suffer in this way endure a different kind of pain than that which is caused by illness or depression—and this pain often ultimately leads to joy because those who endure it are willingly entering into it, as they give up their lives for their Savior.

I've learned that God will actually meet my needs more abundantly and completely when I surrender to Him and His plans and purposes for my life. When I'm tight fisted and do things my way, I don't believe I am as blessed or prosperous.

Maybe depression is hindering you from pursuing, living out or thriving in the fullness of your calling. If so, remember that God's Spirit inside of you is greater than the wounds of your soul, and He can do all things through you, even when it doesn't seem like it. As you obey Him in the little things, you will likely find your spirit being enlarged so that you can function and obey Him in the greater things!

The apostle Paul stated that he had learned the secret of being content in any and every situation (Philippians 4:12). I believe that this is because he walked in great intimacy with God, and wherever He was, He served Him and obeyed Him. Consider that obeying God's will for your life will bring you great contentment, joy and peace, too, not more depression or ungodly suffering!

If your daily life involves doing work or activities that seem meaningless to you, or which go against your values, conscience and/or God-given calling, this may contribute to the depression that you battle. This is because (as I mentioned earlier) when we are out of alignment with God, we will tend to feel discontented and disconnected, because our spirits know that we are either not where we belong, aren't doing what God has called us to do, or aren't doing it with the right attitude.

At the same time, circumstances are usually a fruit, not a root, of depression. This is because circumstances are often an outworking of what we believe about ourselves, others and God, so when we battle fear, self-loathing, shame, self-hatred, hopelessness, helplessness, an unhealthy fear of God (there is a healthy fear of God, but that's not what I'm talking about here) and other emotions related to depression, we will tend to shrink back from living out of our highest potential. Instead, we will create circumstances that align with the lies that we believe about ourselves, rather than taking advantage of those opportunities that reflect the truth of who God has made us to be.

For example, you might avoid pursuing a risky, but fulfilling career out of fear, or refrain from sharing the love of Jesus Christ with others because you don't feel worthy or smart enough. Or maybe you just aren't sure what God's will is for your life, so you play it safe and take on work opportunities that provide a steady income, rather than exploiting the gifts that He has given you by choosing work that is more fulfilling and more in alignment with your calling and who He's made you to be.

We all make decisions that we think will make us safe but we often live unfulfilled in circumstances that we loathe. As another example, maybe you remain in safe but unhealthy relationships or those that God did not ordain for you, because you figure that a relationship with somebody is better than no relationship with anybody and you're scared to be alone, although inwardly you feel like your wings have been clipped.

If you find you derive little joy from your daily work; if you feel like you are just going through the motions of life, or are living a life that isn't true to who you are and what God has called you to do and be, and that includes being in relationships that are not ordained by Him, your spirit may grow anemic and your soul will suffer. You can serve God wherever you are at, and learn to be content even in challenging situations, but you thrive the most when you do what He's called you to do.

Yet again, many of us don't live in the fullness of our calling, because we're scared, don't feel equipped or know the next steps to take, or even realize what we were made for. I've often thought it strange that in our upbringing, most of us are taught about subjects that have little relevance to our lives as adults. What if schools offered courses in life skills, and in discovering your gifts and talents and the purposes of God for your life—just to name a few?

It's no wonder that so many of us finish school and find ourselves graduating high school or college without a clue about who we are or what we've been called to do. We've been taught those subjects that a secular society decided we should learn (unless you went to a religious or private school, which isn't most of us), rather than subjects that have to do with God and real life, and how to cultivate those skills and talents that He has placed within each one of us. Even more importantly, we aren't taught about God's message of salvation and how to share it and the love of Jesus Christ with others. Why is this something we learn at age 30 or 40, or not at all?

Well, never mind! I spent many years trying to discover my life's purpose. Even after I graduated college with a degree in Spanish for Business (yes that was my major!), and before I really knew God, I didn't know what I wanted to do with my life or who I was created to be. So I ended up taking on a job as a flight attendant and traveling the world because I loved to travel. I didn't recognize at the time that God had put that love of travel in me for a reason.

Shortly after I gave my life to Jesus, I was given several prophetic words—which are words from God that came to me through other people—about how God was calling me to be a healing evangelist, and share His gospel, or message, with people in other nations, as well as in my home country. I was delighted, because I had witnessed the suffering of so many people around the world, and really wanted to be a part of seeing them healed, restored and reconciled to God.

I haven't yet fulfilled God's commission for me in its entirety, but I have had the opportunity to go on a few mission trips overseas. Lyme disease prevented me from traveling much for years, but I have since been blessed to be able to minister and share the love of God with people in a handful of Latin American countries, including Cuba, Colombia, Costa Rica and Argentina. I have ministered in churches as well as to the homeless and have even been featured on television on a Miami-based Spanish-speaking health program! I think God has a sense of humor because it seems He has given me more speaking opportunities in my second language than in English, as if to show me that He can use me for anything—including speaking publicly in a language that is more difficult for me than my native English!

I am honored by the ways in which God has used me though, and I hope to be able to continue traveling and ministering to people abroad, as well as at home. Nothing gives me greater joy than to share Jesus Christ with others, pray for their healing, and simply love them with God's love.

If you're thinking, *I have no idea what God made me for, or what I want to do!* I encourage you to spend some time alone with Him, just asking Him and then listening for His reply. If you have asked Him, but aren't sure of the answer, you could ask Him to help you recall the things that you used to enjoy doing in childhood or your early adult life. Your passions and interests can provide clues into what He has created you to do. After all, He puts certain desires and interests in your heart for a reason!

Or, think about what you like to do now. Is it holding babies in a nursery? Helping children to learn math? Painting? Woodworking? Cooking? Taking care of animals?

Planting gardens? Speaking? Encouraging and counseling others? What about politics? Are you entrepreneurial or do you prefer working for others? Ask yourself what interests God has put in your heart and why, and how He wants to use these, along with the natural and supernatural talents and gifts that He's given you, for His Kingdom purposes.

Similarly, you might ask your friends and family what gifts and talents they see in you and what type of work or ministry that they think that you would thrive in. Ask your parents, former caregivers or other family members who know you well, what you used to do that you really loved. Ask God to confirm His Word to you through Scripture, dreams, visions, other people, and circumstances. Ask Him to put people in your path that can help to guide you and align you with your destiny. All of these things can provide valuable insight into what God has created you to be, and what He's called you to do.

Perhaps you know for what you've been made, but you have been afraid to step out into your calling because you believe that you don't have the resources, physical ability, willpower, desire, mental clarity or right connections to get there. Maybe depression keeps you from even getting out of bed, much less going beyond your front door. Maybe you feel helpless and hopeless and that you have nothing to offer others because the reality of who God has made you to be hasn't touched your heart deeply yet. Maybe you don't know what the first, or next step toward your destiny is supposed to be, or you just don't see how you'll ever get from A to Z.

If any of these feelings describe you, know that no matter how inadequate you may feel, or whatever hindrances you may be facing, God has given you unique gifts, abilities and talents to use for His kingdom. Even if you don't know what they are, they are still there, waiting for you to discover them! And while the enemy, the devil, may try to stunt you in your calling, God is greater than every hindrance, roadblock or challenge that you will ever face.

Nonetheless, if you feel lost, I can relate! I used to pray constantly for God to show me what I was supposed to be doing with my life. I was in a quandary since I was nearly incapacitated by Lyme disease. Once, God told me to seek His face, and pursue intimacy with Him, because out of that intimacy I would find the direction in which I needed to go. My passion and the revelation of His plans for my life would be birthed out of His heart and desire for me, and those that He had called me to minister to.

Finally, one day I heard Him say, "I want you to write," and from that, He gave me ideas and began to open doors for me in the writing realm. My Lyme disease blog was a first step into that, which eventually led to many books, but getting to that point was a process. However, I still have many dreams and goals that God has put in my heart to fulfill, and while I don't know how or when those will be fulfilled, I simply seek Him day by day, trusting that He will continue to lead and guide me.

Every great project that God gives you to do starts with baby steps. When I was sick and God told me to write, I almost laughed. My brain could barely pull two sentences together and I didn't know what He wanted me to write. So I just did what came to mind, which was to start a blog to share with others what I was learning about Lyme disease. It was actually fun, if not difficult at times, because I struggled to think. Although my blog didn't get more than about 10 visitors a day at first, after a year there were about 100 visitors per day, and over the next few years, the numbers increased even more. I enjoyed being able to help people with what I wrote.

I knew that God had given me a gift and calling as a writer, and although I didn't know how to fulfill that calling, I gave God something to work with by taking baby steps to use my gift to glorify Him through a simple blog. So just give Him something to work with—if you just give Him an inch, He can take you miles!

God responded in a similar way to my initiative to become involved in healing prayer ministry. Once I learned that it was God's will to heal everyone, I began to look for ways to pray for others, even before I was myself healed. Over time, this resulted in the establishment of a regular prayer conference call group and God giving me a powerful anointing to heal others.

Doing things for others can mitigate depression, when you see the positive effects that your service and life have upon others. Don't serve out of a desire to earn God's favor though, or you will find yourself in a performance-based relationship with Him and burn out. Simply do it because you love Him and people, and because you know that being others-centered is what will bring you the highest level of joy and fulfillment that there is.

Surrendering to God is also a key to knowing His will for your life. It's difficult to hear Him if you are so fixated on your own agenda that you can't hear what He might say to you. Try to release those things that you hold on to with a tight fist—whether ideas, plans, goals, a career or anything else—so that He can sanctify those desires and plans and place His plan and dream for your life into your hands. He cares about your goals, dreams and desires, and most likely put many of them into your heart, but you must release them to Him, for Him to purify and do with as He wishes, in His perfect timing. And be open to the idea that He may have something totally different in mind for you; something which is even bigger and better than what you've dreamed of for yourself!

I encourage you to determine each day to do *just one thing* that will draw you closer toward God's destiny for you, using the gifts and talents that He's given you. That could mean posting a word of encouragement to others on Facebook, researching a class that you've wanted to take, volunteering at a soup kitchen, reaching out to pray for a friend, learning to garden, or taking the next baby step in your chosen career path.

Or, it could simply mean choosing to spend more time with God, committing to a new spiritual discipline, or doing just one new little thing that He's asked you to do—such as thanking Him for the ways in which He's blessed you, or singing a few praise songs to Him in the morning.

Your destiny is likely be revealed to you as a byproduct of your relationship with God, rather than by you trying to figure things out all the time. In fact, you'll probably learn more about who you are and what God has created you to do and be, just by spending time with Him, than by continually brainstorming or using your intellect to assess your life.

Even if you do just one little thing in obedience to God to further your life's calling, such as praying once a week for someone in need, or writing the first page of that new book, you'd be surprised how much of a difference these seemingly small disciplines can make in your life, and how much, over time, they will add up to significant achievements or doors to new opportunities. Remember, God will help you, because He wants to see you happy and living out His dream for you, and He knows that your healing will come, at least in part, as you flourish and blossom in all that He's created you to do and be!

Chapter Seven

Cultivate a Lifestyle that Fosters Wellness

Does your life ever feel imbalanced, with little time, energy or space for God, rest, recreation, and healthy relationships? I believe that God has created us with a desire for all of these things, yet many of us don't have one or more of them in our lives to the extent that God, or we desire. Yet when they are largely absent from our lives, especially healthy relationships, it can create imbalances that can cause or contribute to the depression that we already battle.

Consider this: Jesus was always involved in community and relationship with others. He spent time alone with His Father but He wasn't a loner. He worked, but also took time out to rest and enjoy others. Even God the Father rested, creating the world in six days and resting on the seventh. (Exodus 20:11). While God doesn't technically need rest, I believe that He ceased from His activities in creating the world as an example to us, to take time off, and so that we would take a day off to celebrate Him!

He doesn't want you to live a joyless life of isolation where you do little more than complete your "to do" list daily or overwork, or conversely, lie all day on the sofa with your eyes glued to the television.

At the same time, I realize that depression may cause you to feel apathetic and quench your desire to do much in the first place. Maybe you have to push yourself to get outside the front door to do anything, including going to appointments or work. Maybe you don't even feel like connecting with friends and loved ones, or because of a medical condition, you are physically unable to do so.

Or, perhaps you struggle to find leisure activities that you enjoy, or just want to be alone at home because you feel that people don't understand, love or accept you. Maybe isolation and doing nothing, or conversely, overworking, are easier than finding time and energy to have fun and connect with others, or facing the emotional issues that have caused you to live a imbalanced life.

Maybe you cloak your fears of community and being in relationship with others in rational excuses. Maybe you tell yourself that if you spend too much time with your friends or go out to do fun things, you won't get your work done, and then won't be able to pay your bills. Maybe you tell yourself that you don't need to rest; that life is short and you have work to do, but beneath that seemingly logical excuse is the deep lie that you are unworthy of a happy life, or that your worth is determined by what you do.

Or, perhaps you limit your friendships or interactions with others, because you fear that people won't understand you and your condition and might therefore reject you. After all, nobody wants to be around a sad, depressed (and even sick) person, right?

Consider this: a lot of our decisions that look logical and seem rational to us are really based on fear and lie-based thinking. Yes, there are times in our lives when we might not truly have a lot of time for rest, downtime or energy for friends, family or social gatherings. We may find ourselves in situations where these things become impossible for a season.

There are times when a crisis will demand all of your energy and time, but if you live from crisis to crisis, and your normal life involves little downtime, recreation, fun, rest, or time with God, friends and family, you may find yourself feeling like you are existing, rather than truly living.

In the United States, we highly value productivity and performance, and sometimes view leisure activities or downtime as optional and unimportant, as our society has taught us that our worth comes from what we do, rather than who we are or our identity in Jesus Christ. It's almost a badge of honor to tell people that you're busy. While being busy, in and of itself isn't bad, it can become a problem when work and other obligatory tasks take up all your time and energy, and you have no desire for relationships, rest, social activities or God.

Even if you love your work, or don't work, chances are, you will find depression much easier to overcome when your life includes other things that bring you joy besides work, and that means relationships, rest and rewarding activities. The devil will often lie to you though and tell you that spending time with God or other people doesn't matter, and that you should instead be doing something more productive. You might even feel like your time with God is a waste if you feel unchanged or emotionless after your prayers or quiet time with Him. Yet the purpose of connecting with God isn't just so that He can fill you with positive emotions, but so that you can get to know Him and love Him, just as He loves you.

Maybe you are on the opposite end of the spectrum and have all kinds of free time, but don't feel like doing much, including spending time with others. Maybe you can't. Maybe you're sick or don't have much energy, or you don't know how to get out and be in the world anymore. Or maybe, as I mentioned earlier, fears are holding you back.

As I mentioned earlier, because I was sick for so many years, I lost the ability to do many things that I loved, including outdoor activities that fed my soul, like hiking, skiing and traveling. For years, I felt like a prisoner inside a jail cell as I observed everyone around me participating in life, while I stayed home. At times, I tried to participate in the world around me, but would often be discouraged when my body failed to cooperate and I couldn't keep up with others.

I also battled workaholic tendencies (and admit that I still do!), and for years, spent most of my time either working to make ends meet while I was sick, or doing medical research to discover the next medicine that my body needed. I told myself that I couldn't afford friendships, fun or downtime. Few people understood me, or my battle with Lyme disease and depression, and for a long time, I truly didn't have much time or energy for social events, recreation or fun. I slept a lot and could only function relatively well for a few hours each day.

I also discovered that people generally don't understand chronic illness and depression unless they have had it themselves and can be very unsupportive of the needs and challenges of a person who battles these things, especially when the conditions drag on for years, so for a while, I quietly stopped trying to participate in society.

Time and again, I silently hoped that my loved ones would understand and accommodate my needs, but I found that no amount of explaining, begging, hoping and pleading would change the fact that nobody would "get it until they got it!" It took me a long time to really understand this, and to accept others for their limitations and sometimes very limited ability to love me.

Perhaps you feel the same way. Maybe your loved ones and acquaintances who have never battled depression don't seem to support or understand you, and you've found that it's easier to isolate yourself than to have to ignore quizzical looks or ward off judgmental questions or comments from others.

Regardless of your battle, if you're not in life-giving relationships with other people, or you seldom find yourself with time for God, rest, recreation or activities outside of work, your recovery may be more challenging. In fact, studies have found that social isolation exacerbates depression.[ix]

God created us to be in relationship with one another. Many people in the United States live alone or in isolation and do little with their lives outside of working. Or, they have allowed social media to become a replacement for real life, face-to-face relationships. I don't believe that this is what God intends for us! As I mentioned, God created the world in six days and rested on the seventh, and in the Old Testament He also commanded the Israelites to do the same, by observing the Sabbath, or a day of rest on the seventh day of the week. So there is a Biblical precedent for taking time off for the "three R's": rest, recreation and relationships.

If you're like me, perhaps you've determined at times to be more social with others or take up a new hobby. Maybe you've intended to spend more time relaxing or doing fun things, but fear, busyness, apathy or something else keeps you from doing that and you find long-held patterns difficult to break.

Determination may not be enough if you know that a balanced life is a happy life but you don't know why or how to get there. But it may simply mean making some small but do-able adjustments to your life. First, you may want to ask God what's holding you back from pursuing healthy relationships, fun, rest or whatever it is that's keeping you from living a fulfilling life. If it's a belief, He may need to heal your heart so that you can have the incentive and vision to change some of your daily habits or routine.

Although we have an advocate and helper, the Holy Spirit, who works in us to "will and to do," (Philippians 2:13) the journey toward balance and a better life may require you to do things that are uncomfortable, or which make you feel vulnerable or uneasy in some way. Many good things in life involve risk, doing what's difficult, and getting out of your comfort zone. If you're depressed, you may lack the motivation to even get off the sofa or even out of your home. It's okay—ask the Holy Spirit to help you, and to show you what baby steps you can take that will invite a greater measure of joy into your life and feed your soul and spirit. Ask Him what truly makes your heart sing! Then take a risk to do something differently!

If you're out of touch with what makes your spirit happy and your heart rejoice ask Holy Spirit to show you the things that you used to do that you once enjoyed. Or, perhaps there are things that you've wanted to do, but which you've forgotten about, but can do now. Ask Him how and where you can connect with like-minded people who might enjoy the same activities as you, or who have similar values and interests as you.

When I was really sick, I found that watching You Tube videos about foreign nations and cultures helped me to take the focus off of my pain and gave me hope that I would one day get to travel again.

For you, it might mean cultivating a long-lost hobby or getting involved in a new one. Doing creative activities, like drawing, painting, building, gardening, cooking or photography, is often a good balm for depression, as is spending time in nature and contemplating God's creation.

I believe that we were created for the outdoors. Adam and Eve, the first humans, originally lived in a garden, not a building made by man, so I believe that our spirit, soul and body get fed when we spend time in nature and in the sunshine. Taking walks, or simply sitting on a park bench somewhere contemplating a flower garden, can sometimes do a lot to part the dark clouds. You just need to decide to get out and do it!

Sun also causes your body to produce serotonin, one of your brain's principal mood-enhancing neurotransmitters. Your body then converts serotonin to melatonin at night, encouraging deeper sleep. Many depressed people struggle to sleep, and a good night's rest can often mitigate depression, so I encourage you to get 30-60 minutes of sunshine daily. Your body also produces Vitamin D from sunlight, and Vitamin D additionally plays a powerful role in immune function and mood.

If you battle insomnia, you may find my 2017 E-book, *Beyond a Glass of Milk and a Hot Bath: Advanced Sleep Solutions for Chronic Insomnia,* helpful for you. It is packed with novel, outside-the-box tools for sleep and is based on my recovery from insomnia and over a decade of anti-depressant and sleep medication addiction. For more information, see: ConnieStrasheim.org.

If you're reading all this and thinking, *I don't really enjoy doing anything anymore,* or *I don't really like people,* it may be helpful to ask God why. Maybe your brain and body are so chemically imbalanced that you just can't function without some good nutrition or brain-balancing supplements that will enable you to get up and go. Perhaps your lack of desire is tied to your fears. If so, again, I recommend asking God to show you what those fears are, so that He can heal them, either in your one-on-one time with Him, or with a counselor or trusted friend. Then, ask Him to give you the courage to take baby steps into the world and find those things that will feed your soul and spirit.

One antidote to the fear of rejection, the judgments of others and being in the world, is to determine to have no expectations of people, and simply love and accept them, no matter what they give or don't give to you. To some extent, we all seek to get our needs met through others, but the more that we can enter into a deep, abiding relationship with God, the less that we will expect others to meet our emotional and physical needs, and the less we will be concerned about how others respond to us or what they think of us. This is because our identity will be rooted in Jesus Christ, not others' opinions of us.

God created us to get some of our needs met through other people, but no one person has been designed to carry the burden of all of our needs. That said, if your basic needs for love and affirmation were not adequately met in childhood, and you've not experienced God's love for you in a profound way you may have a stronger tendency to seek to get those needs met through others. Yet again, no person can make up for the love and affection that you never received in childhood. Only God can fill those emotional voids. He may send people into your life to help do that, but your ultimate healing must come through Him.

Anyway, the truth is, we will all be let down at some point in all of our relationships. The question is, how will we respond to the offenses or rejection? Do we give up on people and relationships because they hurt us, or do we forgive those that we love, realize that nobody is perfect, and choose to accept them for who and what they are? In the end, we hurt ourselves more if we allow the rejection or disappointments that we've faced in our relationships to keep us isolated and out of community with others.

God is the only one who will never let us down, leave us nor forsake us, and when we focus upon helping and loving others, as Jesus commanded, without expecting anything in return, He fills us with His love for them. Besides, you may have noticed that the more life and love that God pours into others through you, the more you will find that love coming back to you. It has often been said that if you want friends, be a friend!

If you need emotional support, go to God, and ask Him to be your friend and strongest supporter—He will say yes! Then ask Him, in a spirit of faith, to bring people to you that you can love, as well as people who will love you (which will not always be one and the same), and who will accept you where you are at in your healing journey.

At the same time, it's beneficial to remember that even the strongest and most loving, godly people have their limitations. I have had wonderful friends who, when my struggle became too long and difficult, pulled away from me. So even though you will often hear it said that true friends will stick by you through the hard times, even Jesus' disciples, who loved Him dearly, abandoned him and fled from Him in his darkest hour—right before He was about to be crucified!

All this said, there are godly people out there that will stick by you and who are willing to hold you up through life's difficult storms. You just have to find those people, and prayerfully ask God to connect you with them.

My beloved Bill, whom I met in my late 30s, has been one person who has stood by me and supported me throughout some of the most difficult years that I battled depression. He met me during a time when I was weaning off of benzodiazepines, which I had been addicted to for years—so he didn't get to witness the best of my happy, glowing personality! Nonetheless, he saw the "real" me through my struggles, which is one of the greatest gifts that any of us can give to another. In short, He saw me as Jesus did, which allowed me to be myself with him.

During my most difficult moments of drug withdrawal, I would awaken Bill in the middle of the night and cry on his shoulder. He would console me, encourage me, and pray for me during those times. He didn't just do this once, or twice, but was there for me, day after day, week after week, and year after year.

It was a breath of fresh air and a surprise to find a human being with such a great capacity for love. Not once did his love for me waver. Not once did his opinion of me change, just because my struggle didn't change, and the depression refused to abate. I kept waiting for him to give up on me, to leave me, to realize that I was a hopeless, helpless black cloud in his life, but he refused to see me except through Jesus' eyes, and to Jesus, I was already healed. He saw my potential, not my problems. He saw the light and love of God in me, not my infirmities, and his love for me was patient, kind, generous, selfless and enduring.

I tried to end my relationship with Bill in the beginning, because I thought I was too sick and broken to be in a relationship with anyone, but Bill refused to give up on me, and he proved me wrong in the end!

What's more, God blessed me with the opportunity to serve Bill in the same powerful way that he served me, when, some years later, between 2015-2017, Bill suffered from multiple, life-threatening complications of congestive heart failure, a condition that he had already had for years when we first met. These complications included a heart attack, a TIA and then a stroke, among other issues. He was hospitalized 10 times between 2015-2017, and these were very difficult years for both of us, as well. On several occasions, we didn't know if he would pull through, but he surprised his doctors every time that he did!

The prayers of many people, along with Bill's positive attitude, faith and unwavering trust in God, along with my tenacious love and care for him—indeed, God's love in me— I believe enabled him to be victorious in multiple situations that many others would not have lived through. His life is one of the greatest examples of God's love and miracle working power that I have ever encountered. Love believes all things. Love endures all things. Love heals. Love enables you to get through situations that you might not otherwise survive. And I have discovered through both of our trials that all we need is God's love, working through us, to get through the worst of the worst storms!

I am so thankful that God sent Bill into my life, to teach me how to both give and receive love, but it's sad to me that the kind of love that I have experienced through him is a love that is uncommon in today's world. It shouldn't be, though! We all have the capacity to love as Jesus did, if we simply choose to allow His Spirit to work through us. Yet surrender is a process and sadly, we won't always find friends or family that support us, regardless of what we go through.

In the meantime, you'll find a lot of chains falling off of you if you are able to simply accept that most people live out of their imperfect and unhealed souls. This means that people may treat you and respond to you at times out of their unhealed soul wounds, as well as out of their love for God. Hopefully, their love for God, or the love that others have shown them, will show more in how they treat you, but a person who has not known the love of God, either directly or indirectly through others, cannot adequately love you.

If you are rejected or mistreated though, know that it isn't because you are un-loveable! God already decided you are loveable because He created you for relationship with Him and sent Jesus to die for you and has promised to never leave you nor forsake you. So, if you are mistreated, whether it has to do with you or not, it doesn't matter, because God determines your value, not others, and He loves you and has deemed you worthy of His love and affection.

Remember, even Jesus, who was the greatest embodiment of love to ever walk the earth, was badly mistreated, even by those who claimed to know, love and follow Him. Still, God commands us to love others as He loved and forgave us, so we must choose to do that, even if we don't feel like it. If you're like me, you may find that when you decide to love people, even when your emotions don't align with your choice, it will shift the spiritual atmosphere around you and within you, and you'll end up getting blessed, too. Depression falls away when we love and bless others, no matter how we feel.

Speaking of serving others, did you know that God designed for you to be most fulfilled and at peace when you are serving others? It may not seem that way, and you may be thinking that you're in too much physical or emotional pain to be able to do much for anyone else right now. That may be true, and God may sideline you for a while so that you can simply receive from Him, heal and be refreshed.

But consider this: if you have received Jesus as your Lord and Savior, the very same Spirit that raised Jesus Christ from the dead lives in you, and He wants to love others through you! You have already been made complete in Him and been given all that you need for life and godliness (2 Peter 1:3), whether you feel like it or not. This means that when you are in relationship with Him, your spirit has a great and mighty capacity to love others. So even if your soul doesn't agree, you can trust God to love people through you. In our day-to-day lives, we are called to "re-present" Christ, and you may just find that as you do that, the depression will lift, even if just temporarily.

Sometimes, on the days when I have hosted prayer conference call meetings, I have been attacked with severe depression. Once, I remember sobbing for hours, just minutes before our prayer call was supposed to start, and I said to Bill, "I can't lead the prayer group. I can't pray for 20 people right now. I'm a wreck!"

Bill would gently remind me that it was God's Spirit in me who led the group, and that He would speak the words through me that He wanted me to pray. Sure enough, God always did, and those meetings ended up being some of the best, because I knew that I had to rely on Him to get me through. His power, glory and love would manifest above my sadness, and often, by the end of the prayer meeting, I would be uplifted and encouraged by the lives that were touched during the meeting.

Know that you carry more within you than you might believe. God in you can do exceedingly, abundantly above all that you ask or think (Ephesians 3:20), so simply trust Him, and let Him lead you!

I want to conclude this chapter by encouraging you to ask God what you can do on a daily basis to live a more balanced and joyful existence, right now. It could be something as simple as getting out of the house to walk or go for a swim or taking a bit of time daily to rest.

Don't try to come up with twenty different habits that you think you need to change or presuppose what you need to do. Sometimes, the things that you need to change most in your life aren't those things that you imagine, even if you have dozens of behaviors and habits that you dislike. God may only want you to change one or two things at a time; those "root" issues that will effectuate change at other levels in your life. Anyway, you'll get overwhelmed if you try to make a list of everything that you think you should be doing differently, and then try to change all of those things, especially at once.

Instead, ask God what the most important thing is that He wants to do in your life, right now. Sometimes, we think that we need to change so many aspects of our lives, but there may just be one or two major issues that are triggering joylessness and hopelessness in us and causing us to operate in dysfunction in other areas of life.

For instance, God may tell you that He simply wants you to cultivate a deeper place of rest in Him. He may be unconcerned with your day-to-day activities and simply want to show you how to take time out to be with Him for five or ten minutes here and there throughout the day. Or, He may want to show you how to do the same activities that you've always done, but out of a spirit of rest and peace, rather than out of rushing and anxiety.

Similarly, He may suggest that you take a Pilate's or art class, join a church group, or get a massage once a week. Maybe adding just one new activity to your life will help jumpstart you into a life of greater joy, and in turn spur you on to other things. Keep an open heart and mind about what He may say to you.

Remember, all change starts with baby steps. When you battle depression, you may not have the energy or motivation to do much, anyway. Trust that God knows what you can do, and what you need in your life right now that will heal you. He'll never discourage or overwhelm you, but He may ask you to do something that involves risk or which is uncomfortable for you. Let's face it—most change is uncomfortable for us, even if it's for our good, but most good things in life involve risk and getting out of our comfort zone. God wants the best for you, but He wants you to take His hand, take courage, and trust that He knows best how to lead you in all things!

Chapter Eight

Thrive in Life-Giving Relationships

In the last chapter, I briefly shared about how cultivating life-giving relationships with others can help to free you from depression. God has created us to thrive through relationship with others, but sadly, too many of us are life-depleting or abusive relationships, which can perpetuate, or even cause depression. None of us has perfect relationships with our loved ones, but if you are in a relationship with a close friend, partner, spouse, family member or other loved one whose behaviors bring you down, drain you, or are in some way abusive, and he or she isn't willing to work on the problems in your relationship, consider whether God would want you to continue in that relationship.

We all have imperfect souls, and few of us live out of our spirits all, or even most of the time, but as much as possible, we need to be in life-giving, godly relationships with others. That means cultivating deep, intimate connections with people who love God with all their heart, mind, soul and strength (Mark 12:30) and who aim to love and serve Him and others, above all else. People who are truly surrendered to God will also seek to love and serve you and will have the humility and desire to work on whatever problems come up in their relationship with you. Again, all relationships come with problems and challenges; the goal shouldn't be to find a trouble-free relationship, but to be in relationship with people who love God and are willing to work through problems in a spirit of love, forgiveness and humility.

If you love God and are in a close relationship with someone who doesn't know Him or truly follow Him—and that might include people whose definition of being a follower of Jesus is simply going to church on Sunday, or reciting an "Our Father" every once in a while, or those who just say that they believe in God—you will be what the Bible calls "unequally yoked" with that person.

The apostle Paul, in 2 Corinthians 6:14-15 illustrates this concept. He says to the church of Corinth, "Do not be unequally bound together with unbelievers [do not make mismatched alliances with them, inconsistent with your faith]. For what partnership can righteousness have with lawlessness? Or what fellowship can light have with darkness? What harmony can there be between Christ and Belial (Satan)? Or what does a believer have in common with an unbeliever?"

In other translations, the word "bound together" is translated as "yoked." A yoke was a tool that was used to fasten two animals together, such as oxen. The yoke is associated with servitude, and from Paul's analogy we can infer that, if one person is walking with God and has it as his or her ambition to love God and others, and the other's ambition is to serve his or her selfish desires, then the two will be moving at a different pace, and their partnership will be unproductive and tedious.

If you are unequally yoked with someone, especially a spouse, you may struggle to be as intimate with God as you'd like, or you may find yourself hindered in what God has called you to do. This is because your partner will not be able to support you as you need, may have goals that are at odds with yours, and/or may even resist you. What's more, he or she may discourage you from pursuing relationship with God, either through his or her words, actions or behaviors.

God wants to be first in our lives, and at the center of all of our relationships. He wants us to love everyone, but our close, personal relationships, such as marriage and intimate friendships, will most benefit us and please Him if they are with people who love Him, too. Proverbs 27:17 says, "As iron sharpens iron, so one man sharpens [and influences] another [through discussion]."

This implies that when we spend our time with others who love God, and who live in alignment with His Spirit, we will become "sharpened" in our spirits, and draw closer to God and His ways. Conversely, the Bible says, "Bad company corrupts good morals." (1 Corinthians 15:33). We are always influenced by the company that we keep—for better or worse.

God creates guidelines for our relationships, not to limit us, but to bless us, because our spirits can't soar and we can't grow, and in some cases heal, if we spend most of our time with people who don't know or love God, or with people who live in opposition to His ways. This is because people who don't know and love God tend to be interested in worldly things, while those who love Him have His purposes at the forefront of their life's ambitions and make it their life's goal to love Him and others, as they also love themselves.

Abusive relationships are especially a problem, and can cause or worsen depression, and even cause you to become sick in other ways. If you are in a bad marriage or spend a lot of time with family members that are emotionally, verbally or physically abusive toward you, it may be more difficult for you to get well. God can do anything, but if you're daily insulted, berated, brow beaten, criticized, mistreated or physically assaulted, this can wear at your soul and body.

If you are in an abusive partnership or marriage, you must ask yourself and God how much you truly love yourself and your spouse and if the relationship can be restored. If your marriage or other relationship is hindering your relationship with God and keeping you from living out of the fullness of all that He's created you to be, please do something to change that! Don't fear what your husband, wife, friend, partner or family member will say or do if you decide to obey God. Know that if you are obeying Him, He will take care of you.

When it comes to marriage, the Bible says that God hates divorce (Malachi 2:16), but I don't believe that He would expect anyone to stay in an abusive marriage, especially if it strongly endangers your life or your health. If anything hinders us from relationship with God, He wants us to change our situation so that we can be in uninterrupted fellowship with Him.

I'm not suggesting getting a divorce if you are married to an abusive person, although that may be what God tells you to do. Instead, ask Him and perhaps other wise, godly counselors that you trust, how He wants you to handle things. Most likely He will ask you to first forgive your partner, spouse or whomever it is that has been abusing you, and then teach you how to set new boundaries with that person. He may bring others into your life who will serve as intermediaries in your relationship, and/or who will show you and the other person how you can restore your relationship. Or, He may tell you to simply walk away, especially if your life and/or health are at serious risk.

I know two couples who were once going to call it quits: one, because the husband was unfaithful to his wife, and the other, because the husband was emotionally and physically abusive toward his wife. The wives prayed for God's will to be done, and over time, God moved upon both of the men's hearts so that they eventually repented of their behavior and committed to resolving their issues with their wives. Because they did, and because the women trusted God to heal them, God was able to intervene and powerfully change their lives.

Now, the couple with the unfaithful husband has a worldwide marriage ministry, and the other couple is active in leadership in their local church and helps other couples to restore their relationships. God can do anything, but I don't believe He will expect you to stay in any kind of abusive relationship if He knows the outcome will harm you and your relationship with Him. You can trust Him for that.

If you've been abused, particularly in childhood, and your soul has not been healed, you may be drawn to other abusive people and unhealthy relationships, because research shows that we tend to gravitate toward what's familiar to us. This will especially be true if you have inner vows, bitter root judgments and expectations, and unforgiveness toward those who have harmed or offended you, and your soul has not been sufficiently healed through your relationship with God.

Abuse can damage your self-worth until you know that you are truly and fully forgiven, loved and accepted by God, which can take time. When the abuse occurs in childhood, it can cause you to believe that love is synonymous with mistreatment. If you aren't walking closely in relationship with God, you may miss the signs of an abusive relationship and continue to get into harmful ones until you have been healed, so I encourage you to ask God to give you discernment about all of your relationships, and prayerfully consider whether there is anyone in your life that shouldn't be. Then, work with Him and perhaps also a trusted minister to heal the lie-based beliefs and behaviors in your life that have resulted from the abuse and ask Him to help you to set healthy boundaries in all of your relationships.

Boundaries are important because they help you to know where you end and someone else begins. They teach you what you are responsible and not responsible for, in your life as well as in the lives of your loved ones. Boundaries are designed to protect you from harm and help you to find life- giving relationships.

Co-dependency is one common outcome of a lack of healthy boundaries in relationships. In codependency, one or both people in a relationship take on an inordinate amount of responsibility for the other in an unhealthy way. For instance, they may do things for the other person, but only to control him or her in some way, in an attempt to get their own needs met.

Sometimes, codependency can seem very loving, as in codependent relationships, one person will often completely forsake his or her own needs and desires for the sake of another. The person does this to gain approval, acceptance, affection, security, or a sense of self-worth from helping the other person. Because Jesus tells us to lay down our lives for others, the actions of codependents can outwardly seem very generous and loving.

The problem is that in codependency, people serve their loved ones not for the sake of God or their beloved, but instead, for themselves, because they gain some unhealthy reward for themselves in doing so. In taking on an inordinate amount of responsibility for their loved ones, they often do for them what their loved ones should be doing for themselves, and in so doing end up keeping them in a childlike state.

Often, in co-dependent relationships, one person behaves like a caretaker, while the other is the recipient of the caretaking. Outwardly, the caretaker, who takes on responsibility for the other's needs, may seem generous and godly, while the recipient of the caregiving, may seem irresponsible and selfish. The truth is, both are acting in a childlike manner, because they are seeking to get their needs met through another person in an unhealthy way, rather than through God.

People who were raised in abusive or toxic households often have boundary problems that keep them locked in codependent relationships and/or unhealthy patterns of behavior in their relationships. These relationships can foster depression, because in codependency, neither person is being true to God or themselves through the relationship, and both people are actually harming themselves and the other through selfish behaviors. The love in such relationships is tainted by a need to control the other person, so that they themselves don't feel out of control.

Most of us have struggled to some extent with unhealthy boundaries in our relationships. This is normal. However, if you suspect that there are serious boundary issues in your relationships that are affecting your health, or you are involved with someone in a co-dependent relationship, I highly recommend seeking counseling with a trusted minister. Counselors can help you to identify unhealthy behaviors in your relationships, and teach you how to cultivate new, healthier ones.

I have also found the *Boundaries* book series by Christian counselors Drs. Henry Cloud and John Townsend to be tremendously helpful for helping me to identify unhealthy behaviors in my own relationships, and to avoid those that are toxic. You may want to check them out, too!

Boundaries are a complex topic and what I've shared here is just an introduction to the issue, so again, I strongly encourage you to read the *Boundaries* books to learn more, especially if you suspect that you are in an abusive co-dependent or unhealthy relationship that is making you sick.

In the meantime, if you often find yourself in the role of a caretaker, practice giving your loved ones over to Jesus for Him to take care of. Tell yourself, over and over, that you don't need to control their behavior or their lives, and that you can trust God to work in their lives and help them to do what they need to do, and to become what they need to become.

In the meantime, consider 2 Peter 1:3, which says, "For His divine power has bestowed on us [absolutely] everything necessary for [a dynamic spiritual] life and godliness, through [a] true and personal knowledge of Him who called us by His own glory and excellence."

This means that God's Word and Spirit can give you wisdom and discernment about all things, including your relationships, and how to improve upon, avoid or remove yourself from toxic ones, as well as pursue healthy ones. For this reason, I also highly recommend relying on the Spirit, the Word, and your relationship with God when discerning the people that He wants you to be involved with and using the *Boundaries* books and counsel from godly ministers as adjunct support tools.

I am not advocating that you abandon your friends, spouse and family members if they don't know God, or if you are in a difficult relationship with one or more of them right now. I'm just saying that whenever possible, your primary, closest relationships should bring you closer to God, not pull you further away from Him. If they take you away from Him, then consider what you might do to set healthier boundaries with the people in your life, so that you can be fully healed. I also encourage you to do this because God wants to be your first and most cherished love; your greatest source of strength, wisdom, comfort, provision, peace, and so on. He wants to be your closest friend and your Abba Father! If you lose your relationship with Him, then you can easily lose your way in life.

If your spouse, partner, friends, or family have fallen away from their relationship with God or have never had a relationship with Him in the first place, don't abandon them, but find additional friends who will help to encourage you in your walk and relationship with Him. I say this because I realize that some of you who are reading this are in close relationships with people who don't know God. The good news is that you can still win your loved ones over to Him by your example and His Spirit, who lives in you.

God wants you to have healthy boundaries in your relationships, not because He wants to restrict or limit you, but because He wants to bless you, protect you and keep your heart, mind and body safe. He wants you to love everyone, but you can be held back in your destiny and hindered in your healing and relationship with Him, if the words that you speak to or hear from others daily are poison to your soul; if friends and family don't support your relationship with God or your wellness journey, or if the people that you surround yourself with don't impart life, hope and joy to you by how they treat you or by the words that they speak to you. And vice versa!

Nobody is perfect, and even those of us who deeply love God hurt our loved ones at times with our words and behaviors. There will be times when even those who truly love you, will hurt you. As a general rule though, make it your goal to be with people who love God with all of their heart, mind, soul and strength, and who aim to love others as Jesus loved us.

I want to conclude this chapter by asking you to prayerfully ask God whether you have any difficulties in your close relationships that are contributing to your battle with depression. It doesn't have to be an abusive relationship; rather, it could be a problem in a relationship that's draining the life from you or just dragging you down in some way.

Then, ask God what new boundaries He may want you to set with the person in that relationship, or what He wants you to do to improve the dynamics in the relationship for you and the other person. He may suggest that you see a counselor, to help you identify patterns of behavior that are keeping you and the other person in bondage, and to teach you how to create healthier ways of relating to one another. Or, He may suggest that you end the relationship, if it's a toxic relationship that you weren't meant to be involved in, in the first place.

I know that it can be difficult to change the dynamics in an unhealthy relationship, or end a toxic relationship with someone you love, but you must ask yourself how much you truly want to be well. I urge you to make the decision to love yourself enough to do whatever it takes to heal. I think you'll find that as you do, you'll be better equipped to love others in a healthier way, and that you'll be drawn to more life-giving relationships.

Trust that God knows what's best for you, as well as which people need to be in your life, and which don't, so that you can thrive and be all that He has called you to be, and your loved ones can, too. Because as you choose to let people go; either literally or metaphorically, God can then heal them in His way and they will be more likely to look to Him for their healing and happiness, rather than relying upon you to provide these things for them.

In summary, being in healthy, life-giving relationships can play a key role in helping you to overcome depression. If you don't have at least one friend or family member that you can talk to and spend time with on a regular basis, or any relationships that are life-giving, consider joining a club, church, Meet Up group or other organization where you can spend some time with like-minded people. Even if you don't immediately establish close friendships with the people that you meet in these places, simply connecting with others can still impart life and joy to your spirit. In the meantime, ask God to bring the people that He wants you to be in relationship with into your life, and help you to be a good friend and/or companion to others, so that you can eventually create some closer connections!

Chapter Nine

Heal with Happiness-Promoting Foods

Depression isn't just caused by spiritual or emotional factors, but also biochemical or physiological ones, including genetics, although more commonly, toxins in the environment and chronic infections, especially nowadays. This is because our air, food, water and environment have been heavily polluted in recent years with thousands of toxic chemicals, electromagnetic fields and pathogenic microbes, many of which have increasingly been linked to most modern, chronic degenerative diseases, including depression. As you read this chapter, my hope is that you will discover whether your diet, genetics and/or the environment are playing a role in your battle with depression. You may be surprised at what you learn!

I have researched medicine for many years and interviewed over 100 integrative doctors that treat every chronic condition, from cancer to infectious disease, to mental disorders such as depression and anxiety. From my research and interviews, I have discovered that there are literally many thousands of chemical and electromagnetic toxins, as well as hundreds, if not thousands, of pathogenic microbes in the environment—many of which are making us sick. These toxins can affect literally every organ and system of the body, including the brain and nervous system, and all of us are infected with these toxins and microbes, to varying degrees. In this chapter, I will share with you specifically how contaminated food can cause depression, as well as how the right foods can powerfully affect your recovery from depression!

Once upon a time in history, food healed us, sustained us, and gave us life. But today, food has become a mixed blessing, and only some foods nourish the body, while others contaminate it and make us sick. As I mentioned, much of our food supply has been polluted by a multitude of chemical and microbial toxins, including pesticides and herbicides, artificial hormones, antibiotics, plastics, and other carcinogens that damage the body and cause dysfunction, including mental conditions such as depression.

Food should be medicine for your body. No vitamin supplement, therapy or drug can heal your brain and the rest of your body like food. Food is the fuel upon which your body operates, regenerates and repairs itself. Neither can any supplement can take the place of food, and no manipulating of food can make it better than how God originally created it. To think that we can mess with God's original design for food by altering its DNA, depleting the soil in which it grows of vital nutrients, and adding toxins to it that God didn't create our bodies to process, and not pay a price for it, is naïve.

According to World Life Expectancy, the United States has among the highest incidence of depression and neurological disease in the world, ranking in the top ten for most neurodegenerative diseases including Multiple Sclerosis, Parkinson's and Alzheimer's.[x] However, and as I noted in Chapter One, researchers collaborating with the World Health Organization World Mental Health (WMH) Survey Initiative found that the United States, along with France and the Netherlands, were estimated to have the *highest* percentage of people who battled major depression at least once in their lifetime.[xi] This is despite the fact that the United States spends more money on health per capita than any other nation!

Dietrich Klinghardt, MD, PhD, a renowned integrative medical doctor who specializes in neurological disease, confirms this in my 2016 book, *New Paradigms in Lyme Disease Treatment: 10 Top Doctors Reveal Healing Strategies that Work*. He says, "The results of a study that came out in early 2015 showed that the incidence of death among women with neurological diseases in the United States has increased 663 percent over the past 20 years. Not only that, but the United States has the highest rate of neurological disease in the world, exponentially so. This is caused by the unfortunate combination of this nation's exposure to microbial infections and toxins such as glyphosate and aluminum," [xii] all of which are found in abundance in the food, air and water.

Dr. Klinghardt also says, "There are an estimated 82,000 man-made toxic compounds in our environment. If appropriate detection methods are used, all of these compounds can be found in our bodies. We all are contaminated with huge amounts of toxins, and it's the unhealthy 'terrain' of our bodies that sets the stage for us to become sick from pathogenic microbes and other factors."[xiii]

Environmental toxins, especially aluminum and other heavy metals like mercury, as well as pathogenic microbes that are found in our food and water, can cause or contribute to depression, in addition to other neurological conditions such as Alzheimer's, Parkinson's, Lyme disease, chronic fatigue syndrome, and Multiple Sclerosis. Hundreds, if not thousands of studies that have been published on government databases such as PubMed.org substantiate this, as well as many integrative and naturopathic doctors' experiences with their patients.

For instance, many studies reveal a strong link between aluminum toxicity and Alzheimer's disease. [xivxvxvi] Toxins and microbes inflame the brain, and inflammation, which I will discuss more about later, is in itself a major cause of depression.

According to Dr. Klinghardt, who travels and teaches worldwide, European countries have historically used fewer toxic pesticides and herbicides on their crops than the United States. [xvii] Consequently, these countries have a lower incidence of neurological conditions, since pesticides and herbicides have been linked to neurological disease, including depression.

For instance, a study published in July 2017 in the journal *Neurotoxicology* showed that people in Korea exposed to pesticides had significantly higher rates of depression. [xviii] The authors of the study also note that pesticides, in general, have been associated with a higher incidence of mental disorders.

Of course, the United States may have higher rates of depression and other neurological diseases for other reasons, too. In any case, and according to Dr. Klinghardt, the environment in Germany, Austria, Italy and Hungary is much cleaner than that of the United States, and the food in Germany is richer in minerals, which may partially account for a mentally healthier population.[xix]

The toxins found in our food, air and water can contribute to or cause depression for a variety of reasons. First, as I just mentioned, they cause brain and nervous system inflammation. Secondly, they damage neurons and beneficial bacteria in the brain and gut where most neurotransmitters are made, as well as the gut lining itself. When the gut is damaged, this can lead to leaky gut syndrome, a condition in which undigested food particles pass through the damaged gut walls and enter the bloodstream, where they trigger systemic inflammation. Toxins also damage the body's enzyme systems and the liver's ability to synthesize, break down and detoxify proteins, including brain chemicals—and that's all just for starters.

In addition, in the United States, modern farming practices have depleted the soil of micronutrients. Studies show that vegetables and fruits contain just 30-50% of the nutrients that they did just 50 years ago. An article published in *Scientific American* states, "A landmark study on the topic by Donald Davis and his team of researchers from the University of Texas (UT) at Austin's Department of Chemistry and Biochemistry was published in December 2004 in the *Journal of the American College of Nutrition.* They studied U.S. Department of Agriculture nutritional data from both 1950 and 1999 for 43 different vegetables and fruits, finding "reliable declines" in the amount of protein, calcium, phosphorus, iron, riboflavin (vitamin B2) and vitamin C over the past half century. Davis and his colleagues chalk up this declining nutritional content to the preponderance of agricultural practices designed to improve traits (size, growth rate, pest resistance) other than nutrition."[xx]

Your body requires and utilizes a broad spectrum of vitamins, minerals, amino acids and essential fatty acids for brain function and nervous system health. When you lack the appropriate amounts of certain minerals, vitamins or other essential nutrients, such as amino acids—which are the building blocks of neurons and neurotransmitters—it is difficult for your brain to function properly. It is beyond the scope of this book to describe the role of every nutrient in mental health, although I will share about some important ones in Chapter Eight.

In the meantime, know that your body, brain and mind function optimally when you give them the nutrition that they need, whether through food or supplements. Later in this book, I'll share with you how you can discover what nutrients your body needs for optimal mental health and how to make up for any deficiencies.

Another problem with the food supply in the United States is that conventionally raised farm animals, especially cows and chickens, are fed a non-native diet; that is, foods that their bodies weren't designed to consume. For cows, this means corn and animal byproducts. In addition, these animals are given growth hormones to grow at an abnormally fast rate and are then injected with antibiotics to counter the infections that result from their poor diet, abnormal growth rate and inhumane living conditions, since most of these animals spend their lives in crowded pens or feedlots.

The growth hormones, antibiotics and toxins that the animals consume get transferred to your body when you eat their meat, and can destroy your gut flora, create perforations in your small intestine that cause leaky gut, and cause de-regulation of your endocrine, nervous and immune systems. Many neurotransmitters are actually made in your gut, not just your brain, and the beneficial bacteria there play a vital role in your brain and immune function, in addition to your digestion, so it's crucial to keep your gut healthy! Hormonal de-regulation is another major cause of depression, which I discuss more in depth later in this book.

Finally, due to clever marketing schemes, many of us are consuming foods that we have been taught are healthy for us but which really are not. Labels like "low fat," "enriched with Vitamin X," "natural," and "low calorie," have fooled some of us into believing that just because a label touts some health benefit, then that food must be good for us.

But consider this; foods that support a healthy mood and body don't need advertising. For instance, take granola bars or yogurt, which are often marketed as health foods, but which usually contain high amounts of sugar and/or artificial ingredients. Such foods are inflammatory and may contribute to depression.

I'll tell you a secret: the only foods that are truly life, health and happiness promoting are those which God made and which have been unadulterated by man. They are things that your great-grandmother would recognize as food. Healthy food doesn't come in a box or a can. It comes from one of four places: directly from the ground, the sea, a plant or an animal!

Foods that contain artificial preservatives, those which are extensively processed (meaning, they contain more than five ingredients on their ingredients label!) or which are found in a box or can are generally unhealthy for you and may cause inflammation and chemical imbalances that cause or exacerbate depression.

This means that at least half of what's found in your conventional supermarket can make you sick and sad! The remaining half, which includes organic produce, nuts and seeds, and animal protein, is usually found around the perimeter of the supermarket, so shop there and avoid the middle! If that sounds extreme, consider that what we've done to our food supply is extreme and why, in the United States and elsewhere, we are facing an epidemic of depression and neurological disease.

Renowned integrative doctor Keith Scott Mumby, MD shared in my 2011 book *Defeat Cancer: 15 Doctors of Integrative and Naturopathic Medicine Tell You How* a story about how food allergies made one of his young patients murderously violent. When Dr. Mumby convinced the youth to stop eating a particular type of food that was making him sick, the youth calmed down and his mood stabilized.[xxi] Food can powerfully influence your mood!

This is actually wonderful news for some of you who are reading this, because it means that eating the right foods has the potential to do more for your physical, mental and emotional wellbeing than any drug or other therapy for depression. Food is that powerful. If you don't believe me, just try following the guidelines outlined in this chapter for a month or two and see how you feel. Even if you know that your depression is caused principally by emotional, genetic or spiritual factors, balancing your brain and body with life-giving foods can make a world of difference in how you feel.

How to Find Life-Giving and Mood-Promoting Foods

There are so many diets out there and so much conflicting advice about which foods are healthy and which aren't, that it can be hard to know what foods will best help you to recover from depression and any other health conditions that you may be battling. In this section, I'll share some dietary guidelines that I've found to be beneficial for a majority of people and which can help you determine what to eat daily for optimal wellness.

First, as I mentioned, you'll find most life and mood-promoting foods around the perimeter of your local supermarket. This is where all the natural, or "real" food, such as fruits, vegetables and animal proteins such as eggs, chicken, beef and turkey are stocked. You'll want to purchase most of your food here. Later, I will share with you more specifically which foods are packed with mood, mind and energy-promoting nutrients.

Even better, go to your local organic farmer's market, where you can find local produce that's likely to be more nutrient-rich than many of the foods that are found in your grocery store. This is because not all grocery store produce is local and is often shipped across many states and/or countries, which means that it has to be picked prematurely so that it doesn't spoil by the time it reaches the store. Premature fruits and vegetables that don't have a chance to ripen to maturity are often nutrient-deficient. So eat local food, whenever you can. By doing this, you'll also reduce your "carbon footprint" as shipping food long distances uses up a tremendous amount of natural resources and increases environmental pollution.

Some non-gluten grains, legumes and other foods that are typically found in the middle sections of the supermarket are sometimes healthy, depending on the overall condition of your health. If you have a chronic, neurodegenerative disease like I did, for instance, you may find it best to eliminate all legumes and grains from your diet, because these can exacerbate damage in your gut, if your gut health is already compromised, and cause systemic inflammation. Remember, whatever affects your gut will also affect your brain and your mood.

In general, the categories of food that most researchers and doctors I know have found to be best for promoting a happy mood and healthy body in their patients include: organic vegetables, fruits, and nuts; organic meat and other animal protein products from pasture-raised animals, and healthy oils such as coconut and olive oil. Some healthy grains and legumes, and a few organic dairy products may fall into this category as well, again, depending upon your overall health.

Secondly, make sure that your animal protein, especially beef, chicken, pork and eggs, come only from pasture-raised animals that have not been fed a non-native diet, hormones and antibiotics. Unfortunately, animal protein that is labeled "organic, free-range" and "fed a vegetarian diet" is not necessarily healthy (vegetables and fruits labeled organic are okay though) because many "free range" animals only spend about five minutes outside their crowded pens daily, rather than a majority of their lives outdoors, as they should. These animals, while they may not be given antibiotics or hormones, are often fed a non-native diet of genetically modified corn and soy, and grains that contain arsenic, all of which have been found to be highly allergenic and toxic to most people.

Instead, look for labels on chicken and eggs that read "pasture-raised" in addition to antibiotic and hormone free. For beef, look for "100% grass-fed and grass-finished" as beef can legally be called organic and grass-fed, even if the cows were fed a non-native diet of corn during the last part of their life!

Pasture-raised poultry and 100% grass-fed beef may be challenging to find in some supermarkets, but you can often find them at smaller organic farms, and/or order them online from companies such as US Wellness Meats: USWellnessMeats.com. They are more expensive, but so are being depressed or sick! If you don't have access to this kind of meat, at least choose organic antibiotic and hormone-free products, whenever possible.

If these guidelines seem extreme, consider that animals that are fed a non-native diet have dangerous chemicals such as arsenic and pesticides in their feed, which get into your body, damage your gut, and create a setup for inflammation and depression.

Also, don't be fooled by labels that read: "natural beef" or "natural chicken." This means nothing. Of course, the animal is natural — didn't God make it? Rather, the packaging label should read, "pasture-raised, antibiotic (rBGH), and hormone-free."

Organic vegetables and fruits, and the meat from pasture-raised animals are generally cleaner and of a higher quality than that which comes from conventionally raised produce and animals. What's more, pasture-raised animals are given a more humane life. This is truly the only real healthy food anymore in the United States. I feel strongly about the necessity of eating clean food, because I have seen the studies and interviewed the researchers and doctors that have witnessed firsthand how the toxins in non-organic foods cause disease. I've also experienced much greater wellbeing myself whenever I eat clean food.

Again, I know that organic food can be expensive but, in the end, you may want to consider how badly you want to be well. I found a way to afford organic food, even when I lived on Social Security Disability income and food stamps. I shopped at co-ops, ate less, and bought sale items. God made a way because I asked Him to and I believed that He would. If the demand for real food in this country increases, over time it should become less expensive.

In addition, please avoid genetically modified foods (GMOs), which studies have shown to be difficult for the body to digest and to contain pesticides. GMO's have been linked to autoimmune disease, cancer, chronic inflammation and other health problems. A study entitled "Genetically Engineered Crops, Glyphosate and the Deterioration of Health in the United States of America" which was published in *The Journal of Organic Systems* in 2014 shows significant correlations between GMOs and 22 diseases.[xxii]

God can heal you supernaturally and through your relationship with Him, but if you are filling your body daily with lots of toxic chemicals or artificial food, it may be more difficult to maintain that healing. If that seems far-fetched, consider whether God created the human body to consume fertilizer, heavy metals, chemicals, pesticides, plastics, antibiotics and artificial hormones on a daily basis. We all have a different level of tolerance to toxins, and God can sustain you supernaturally in spite of what you eat, but most of us can't consume an unlimited amount of harmful chemicals without repercussions. It's just a question of how much your body can handle before symptoms manifest. Anyway, in the end, you won't know how much better you can feel unless you try eating clean, unprocessed food!

If you truly can't afford organic food, you can ask God to bless your food and He may protect your body from the effects of any contaminants that are in it. Jesus says of His followers in Mark 16:18, "if they drink anything deadly, it will not hurt them." I believe that this can apply to our food, too, but I don't know anyone who lives entirely above the natural realm yet and has been able to live totally unaffected by the environment. But according to your faith in God's power may it be done unto you! (Matthew 9:29).

I also think we can tempt God by intentionally consuming foods on a regular basis that we know are harmful for us. Many people in the United States are sick, overweight and depressed because they are consuming chemical poisons daily. The chemicals that are sprayed on produce, for instance, have been shown in studies to be neurotoxic. Neurotoxins poison your brain and nervous system and can lead to depression, anxiety and other neurodegenerative conditions.

My faith has allowed me to eat only those things that I know are healthy for me, and until God's people and the church are healthier than the rest of society because we have learned to live supernaturally in divine health, I think it is wise to take care of God's temple that is our body by eating real, clean food.

Thankfully, organic and pasture-raised food is becoming more affordable, as more people are realizing the benefits— indeed the necessity—of consuming clean, unadulterated food. More affordable health food stores are cropping up to compete with the more expensive ones. Where I currently reside in the Dallas area, Central Market provides less expensive, decent quality organic food. If you live in a house or have a patio where you can grow a little garden, this is one way to get nutrient-rich organic veggies. In *Foods that Fit a Unique You,* a book that I co-authored with world-renowned integrative medical doctor, Lee Cowden, MD, Dr. Cowden and I share some simple tips for how you can do that.

The first humans, Adam and Eve, lived in a garden and ate the food that was found there, which was all basically plant-based. In Genesis 1:29, God says to them, "Behold, I have given you every plant yielding seed that is on the surface of the entire earth, and every tree which has fruit yielding seed; it shall be food for you."

Incidentally, many doctors that I have interviewed recommend a vegetable-based diet to their really sick patients. This is because vegetables are the one category of food that has been deemed by the holistic medical community to be healthy for most everyone, with the exception of some genetically modified vegetables like corn and potatoes, and nightshade vegetables such as tomatoes and eggplant. These foods can be problematic for people with allergies or other chronic health conditions.

Beyond that, God created us to consume food in its natural state, whether fruits, vegetables, nuts, grains, legumes or animal protein. At the same time, not everyone thrives on exactly the same diet, even if those foods are generally deemed to be healthy. This is because we are all unique, and because many of us nowadays have leaky gut syndrome and food allergies, it is wise for us to avoid foods that can exacerbate those conditions.

In *Foods that Fit a Unique You,* Dr. Cowden and I share a list of criteria that you can use to determine whether a particular food is healthy for you. This list is based on Dr. Cowden's experience with thousands of chronically ill and depressed patients, and my personal experience and over 10 years of research in nutrition.

First and foremost, we ask, how do you feel after you eat a particular food? Does it make you energetic, tired, grumpy or apathetic? You shouldn't be tired or grumpy after you eat! This is a sign that you either gave your body something that it didn't want, or that you ate too much. Pay attention to how foods make you feel, as this may be the single best indicator of whether a food is life giving for you. Your body knows best!

Now, depression can cause carbohydrate cravings because carbohydrates temporarily raise serotonin, which is a mood-enhancing chemical that your body needs. The problem is that most carbohydrates that do this are not really healthy for you in other ways. There are better ways to raise your serotonin than with cereal, cookies, pastries, pasta and other unhealthy high carbohydrate foods. So, if you are tempted to indulge in these foods on a regular basis, I encourage you to resist, as eating unhealthy carbohydrate foods can, as a side effect, cause inflammation and over the long run, make depression worse.

Secondly, Dr. Cowden advocates testing your pulse immediately after you eat. If you find that it's elevated by more than 15 beats per minute that can be a sign that you just ate something you were allergic to or which your body did not like. Above all things, you want to avoid food allergies, as these, by themselves, can cause depression, since allergies increase inflammation in the brain and the rest of the body.

How do you know if you are allergic to a particular food? Well, unless you ate a large meal, if you are tired, lethargic, brain fogged or grumpy within an hour or two after you eat, or your pulse accelerates shortly after a meal, it is likely that you ate something that you were allergic to or are at least sensitive to. In the short term, that may not be a big deal, but having an allergic reaction to food every time you eat, over time, can cause or worsen depression. Of course, you may find that it's okay to indulge in a tasty pastry or other treat every once in a while, but I don't recommend doing it daily.

Testing Your Body's pH

Another fantastic way to discover the foods that will make you feel your best is to test your saliva pH. This is easy to do and later in this section I will share with you how you can do that. Your pH is a measure of your body's level of acidity or alkalinity. When your saliva pH is less than 7, your body is said to be acidic; when it is greater than 7, it is alkaline. You want your pH to be balanced: neither too acidic nor too alkaline. When it's balanced, you will feel your best.

So, if by nature you are a meat-lover, and you feel good when you eat meat, then your body is more likely to come into better pH balance when you include some meat into your diet. Conversely, if you are acidic and feel poorly when you eat meat, it may be because the meat is making you too acidic. In that case, you would fare better on a diet that is higher in fruits and veggies.

Of course, there are some foods that will make most of us pH imbalanced—such as sugar, extensively processed foods and any other food that's an allergen to the body. Balancing your pH is crucial for healing from depression and any other health condition that you may be battling. Many problems occur whenever your pH is imbalanced. For instance, whenever you are too acidic, your cells cannot properly assimilate nutrients or dispose of metabolic waste, and your body's chemical reactions and electrical responses will be abnormal.

In addition, your body uses its mineral stores to bind, neutralize and remove the excess acid, as acid is dangerous to the body and damages its cells. This, in turn, causes mineral deficiencies, which can contribute to depression and other health problems. Numerous health problems are associated with pH imbalance.

Finally, your body's pH is not only affected by the foods you eat, but also by stress. Managing stress and treating any chronic health conditions will help to balance your pH, as will eating foods that are appropriate for your unique body chemistry.

Note: The following excerpt is taken from Foods that Fit a Unique You, by Connie Strasheim and W. Lee Cowden, MD. @ ACIM Press, 2014.
To learn more, see: ConnieStrasheim.org/books

PH testing is simple. To measure your saliva pH,simply purchase pH-testing strips from an online retailer. A few health food stores may also carry these strips. Make sure that the pH paper that you purchase has a measurement range of 5.5 to 8.0 pH in 0.2 pH increments.

After you eat a meal, brush and floss your teeth thoroughly, then wait four to eight hours after that meal before testing your saliva pH. You'll also want to avoid drinking any water for at least an hour prior to testing.

To do the test, spit three times into the sink. Then spit onto a small strip of the pH paper. After about 15 seconds, the pH paper will have turned a shade of yellow, green or blue, depending on what your saliva pH is. A color-coded chart that corresponds to a set of numbers on the pH strip container will reveal to you whether your pH is too alkaline, acidic or balanced.

If it is too acidic (this is the most common response), consider which of the foods in the meal that you last ate is most likely to be causing the acidity. If you don't know, then consume each of those foods in the meal separately, one at a time, to discern your response to each.

It's best to measure your pH four to five hours after you eat most types of food, except for beef, bison, lamb and other heavy animal proteins, which take longer to digest. It's best to test your pH approximately eight hours after consuming the latter meats.

To find out what your body's baseline pH is, test your pH first thing in the morning, ideally after fasting for 12 hours overnight, and before eating or drinking anything that day. This reading will give you an idea of your overall pH.

The pH test is one way to fine-tune your diet and is a great way to find out whether you are on track with what you are eating. I can provide you with guidelines for how to eat well, but the results you get with pH testing are one way to confirm whether those guidelines are appropriate for you. Ideally, you want your saliva pH reading to be between 6.8 and 7.2. If it is lower, then that means that you are too acidic. If it is above 7.2, then you are too alkaline.

Since your pH is also influenced by stress, I also recommend evaluating any sources of major stress in your life and asking God to help you find ways to eliminate those.

Following are more general guidelines and food lists for healthy eating, which Dr. Cowden and I have found to be mood and health-promoting for a majority of people, and which can help mitigate the symptoms of many health conditions, including depression.

Note: *Parts of the following excerpts are taken from W. Lee Cowden MD's and my book, Foods that Fit a Unique You. @ ACIM Press, 2014. To learn more, see: ConnieStrasheim.org/books.*

Just about every diet book out there advocates eating vegetables. And in fact, veggies are good for most everyone, with few exceptions. They are a rich source of carbohydrates, which provide energy to your cells. Most are rich in beta-carotene (which is converted by your body into Vitamin A), B-vitamins, Vitamins C, K and dietary minerals such as calcium, magnesium, potassium, and iron. Your body uses B-vitamins and minerals to create neurotransmitters, so these nutrients play a crucial role in mood, brain and gut health.

Additionally, vegetables contain high levels of antioxidants, which your body uses to scavenge DNA-damaging free radical chemicals in the bloodstream that can lead to cellular destruction and inflammation, and consequently, depression. Many vegetables also contain fiber, which is necessary for healthy gastrointestinal function. If you'll recall, I mentioned earlier that gut health is intimately tied to brain health and mood. Vegetables also protect your body against a wide variety of illnesses and health conditions, including cancer, diabetes, and kidney stones.

Non-starchy vegetables, which include green veggies such as all lettuces, spinach, Bok Choy, arugula, kale, endive, parsley, asparagus, broccoli, zucchini, green beans and Brussels sprouts, as well as cabbage, summer squash, onions and garlic, are especially well-tolerated by a majority of people.

While nightshade vegetables are nutrient-rich, they cause inflammation in some people. Common nightshade vegetables include: white potatoes, tomatoes, eggplant and peppers (hot and sweet). These veggies contain a substance called alkaloids that can negatively impact nerve, muscle and digestive function, and cause inflammation, especially in people with certain chronic health conditions, such as fibromyalgia, chronic fatigue syndrome, Lyme disease, arthritis, colitis, and autoimmune disease. If you battle depression that's linked to another chronic health condition, you may want to avoid nightshades.

In general, however, organic vegetables are among the most nutritious, health-promoting foods we can eat. I encourage you to include multiple servings daily of any of the following into your diet:

- Artichoke
- Arugula
- Bok Choy
- Broccoli
- Brussels sprouts
- Cabbage
- Carrots
- Celery
- Collard greens
- Cucumbers

- Garlic
- Green onions
- Endive
- Kale
- Leeks
- Lettuce
- Mustard greens
- Onions
- Parsley
- Radish
- Scallions
- Seaweed
- Spinach
- Sprouts
- String beans
- Summer squash
- Swiss chard
- Watercress
- Zucchini

If you don't have another serious health condition, especially a neurological or autoimmune disease, or diabetes, you may also be able to include some starchy and nightshade vegetables into your diet, such as:

- Beet (roots)
- Bell (and other peppers)
- Eggplant
- Mushrooms

- Parsnips (roots)
- Red potatoes
- Sweet potatoes
- Tomatoes
- Winter squash/pumpkin
- Yucca
- Yams

Consume Clean, Pasture-Raised Animal Protein

Sufficient protein intake is vital for overcoming depression. Neurons, neurotransmitters and other physical structures in the brain, gut and nervous system are made from protein, and some of us don't get enough of it. Clean, organic animal protein, in particular, is an important staple of a healthful, well-rounded diet. Most of us feel and function at our best when our daily meals include modest, palm-sized portions of healthy animal protein, including pasture-raised chicken and eggs; grass-fed, non-GMO beef; wild salmon, sardines, anchovies and other small fish; lamb, ostrich, turkey, Cornish game hen, buffalo, elk, bison and other game meat.

It's also important to consume the meat of pasture-raised animals because it contains more health-promoting omega-3 essential fatty acids than conventionally processed meat. Your body uses omega-3 acids to make brain tissue and cell membranes. The most prevalent fatty acid in the brain is called DHA. It is found in pasture-raised animals as well as in fish and is important for normal brain function. If you don't eat much animal protein, you'll want to take DHA as a supplement, to ensure that your brain gets the nutrition that it needs. I recommend Nordic Naturals' fish oil products, which contain DHA. For more information, see: NordicNaturals.com.

Organic Fruits

Organic fruits are rich in vitamins, minerals, micronutrients, fiber and antioxidants, and provide energy and health to your body in a variety of ways. Most fruits boost the immune system because of their high vitamin content, particularly Vitamin C. The antioxidants in fruit help to remove DNA-damaging free radicals from your body that can contribute to depression and other conditions. In addition, they lower unhealthy cholesterol, promote healthy digestion, and protect your body against a multitude of ailments.

Most people can consume at least a modest amount of fruit, although if you are hypoglycemic or pre-diabetic (which is a lot of us!), you'll want to avoid fruits that contain high amounts of natural sugar, such as bananas, grapes and melons, which spike the blood sugar and cause your pancreas to release high amounts of insulin. Instead, you will likely feel better if you stick to fruits with a lower natural sugar content, such as avocados, apricots, pears, apples, berries, grapefruit, lemons and limes. If you have another neurological condition or diabetes in addition to depression, such as multiple sclerosis, Amyotrophic Lateral Sclerosis (ALS), Parkinson's or Lyme disease, you may want to avoid fruit entirely, as even low amounts of natural sugars can sometimes aggravate symptoms of neurodegenerative disease.

You may also want to avoid fruit juice, since it causes blood sugar spikes that can lead to hypoglycemia, inflammation and insulin resistance, all of which have also been linked to depression, in addition to diabetes, metabolic syndrome and other conditions.

Organic Nuts and Seeds

Organic nuts and seeds are an important source of healthy fat and protein for most of us (except for peanuts, which almost always contain mold) and are used by the body as building blocks for hormones, neurotransmitters, organs and other tissue. Most nuts and seeds contain high amounts of fiber, as well as mood-promoting vitamins, amino and minerals, especially magnesium, which plays a role in over 300 enzymatic reactions. Pumpkin seeds are especially rich in tryptophan, a mood promoting amino acid that the body uses to make serotonin. Studies have also shown nuts to protect against cardiovascular disease, and when eaten in moderation, they are a healthful replacement for sugary snacks.

Some of the most nutrient-rich nuts and seeds include: organic walnuts, almonds, Brazil nuts, pine nuts, and pecans, as well as flaxseed, and sunflower, pumpkin, and sesame seeds. Nut and seed butters which don't contain sugar or other additives are likewise healthful.

Non-Gluten Grains and Legumes

Years ago, bread was good for you. Indeed, the Bible indicates that grains were once a healthful, desirable type of food, but now, many people are grain and gluten-intolerant due to the overabundance of gluten in wheat and other grain products, and the prevalence of leaky gut syndrome in the population.

In addition, most wheat, especially in the United States, has been genetically modified and engineered to contain pesticides. You ingest these pesticides whenever you consume bread or other wheat-containing products. The pesticides then damage your gut, cause food allergies, brain inflammation and—you guessed it—depression, among other symptoms.

Some people can still tolerate modest amounts of gluten-containing grains, but as a general rule, more of us than not will do better eating less of this type of food than the others that we've mentioned so far. And here's more news for you—research shows that grains and gluten are the number one food-related cause of depression,[xxiii] so if you haven't tried completely removing grains, at least gluten-based ones, from your diet to see how it affects your wellbeing, I recommend giving it a try for a month or two.

Even if you don't feel badly after eating a slice of bread or bowl of pasta, you are likely to feel more energetic and fare better on a grain-less diet, or at least a diet of tasty, healthy non-gluten grains, which include things such as quinoa, amaranth, millet, spelt and white and brown rice.

Amaranth, which was originally cultivated by the Aztec people of Mexico, is a grain that contains all of the amino acids or protein building blocks that are essential for health. Quinoa, which was originally cultivated by the Inca people of South America, is especially healthful. It isn't a true grain, but rather, a seed that also contains all of the essential amino acids for protein-building, as well as higher levels of protein than any other grain or seed.

Most health food stores sell flours, pastas, breads and other products that are made from a variety of non-gluten grains, nuts and seeds, and which are just as tasty as gluten-containing grains.

Legumes, such as lima, black, kidney and other types of beans; black-eyed peas, lentils, and chickpeas, are also healthy foods for many people, but, like grains, they are best consumed in moderation. Legumes are another type of food that, when eaten in excess, can contribute to mood disorders. Experiment with these to see what makes you feel best!

Organic Goat/Sheep Milk Cheese

Conventionally processed cow milk products are another major source of inflammation; they contain antibiotics, artificial growth hormones, pesticides and many other inflammatory substances, and can also affect your mood and physical health. In addition, cow's milk products are difficult for many people to digest.

If you love dairy, consider exchanging your cow's milk products for organic goat and sheep milk products, especially raw cheese, kefir and sugar and chemical-free yogurt, which contain beneficial bacteria that aid in immune function, as well as brain and gastrointestinal health. These can be healthful sources of protein and are a tasty addition to the diet. Raw dairy products can be obtained at raw dairy farms; they are not available in most grocery stores. However, like grains, dairy products can sometimes contribute to depression, so you may want to remove all dairy products from your diet for a month, to see if you notice a positive change in how you feel. Christiane Northrup, MD, author of *Women's Bodies, Women's Wisdom* has observed that her patients who removed all dairy foods from their diet had fewer symptoms of PMS, including depression.[xxiv]

In general, most people with neurological conditions feel best on a diet that includes greater amounts of fruits, vegetables, healthy nuts, seeds, oils and meat, and lesser amounts of grains, legumes, milk products and of course, processed foods that contain artificial ingredients! Yet again, everyone is different, so I encourage you to experiment and try out the different types of healthful foods that I describe in this chapter, to see how you feel, eliminating all others that may be harmful to your health. Then test your pH after you consume each food, to see if it aligns with your choices. To learn more about how to find foods that fit your unique chemistry, I encourage you to check out Dr. Cowden's and my book, *Foods that Fit a Unique You.*

Plain Organic Yogurt and Other Probiotic Foods

Many brands and types of yogurt fill our grocery store shelves, and I hate to break it to you but—once again, many of these products cause inflammation. Most yogurts, even those which are organic, low-fat, and labeled "natural" contain sugar or artificial sweeteners and an abundance of unhealthy chemicals to preserve them; are made from unhealthy cow's milk, and have been stripped of valuable nutrients, especially probiotic bacteria, because they are pasteurized and homogenized.

Nonetheless, some yogurt products can be a valuable source of protein, as well as minerals such as magnesium and calcium, and immune-enhancing probiotics, or immune-supportive bacteria, which you need for a healthy gastrointestinal tract, immune system and brain. In most cases, these bacteria are stripped from the yogurt during pasteurization and replenished afterwards, but you may still derive some benefit from consuming them.

Raw yogurt is the most health promoting, because it isn't pasteurized and therefore contains all of its original beneficial bacteria and enzymes. Raw yogurt isn't sold in grocery stores, however. You'll need to make it yourself or obtain it from a raw dairy farm. If you do an Internet search and input the term: "raw dairy farm" into the search engine box, along with your city and/or state, you are likely to find farms in your area that sell raw dairy products. Similarly, instructions for how to make homemade yogurt can easily be found on the Internet on websites such as: MakeYourOwnYogurt.com.

Kimchi

Kimchi is a flavorful and healthy fermented Korean food that contains immune-supportive friendly bacteria that help to remove pathogenic microbes that can contribute to a damaged gut, and consequently, an inflamed brain and nervous system.

A healthy human gut has approximately 500 to 1,000 types of friendly bacteria. However, if you have taken antibiotics or routinely consume conventionally processed beef and/or chicken (which are given lots of antibiotics), your gut's bacterial population has likely been dramatically reduced, since antibiotics strip the gut of healthy bacteria. These bacteria are your body's first line of defense against viruses, bacteria, parasites and other pathogens, which enter your gut through your air, food and water, so you want to keep as many of them as possible alive and intact!

If you don't have enough friendly bacteria in your gastrointestinal tract, you will be more susceptible to developing a leaky gut caused by infections and toxins, and your body won't process nutrients as effectively. This leads to nutrient deficiencies and inflammation, and with that, depression. In addition, most of your neurotransmitters are produced in your gut, so a healthy gut equates to a healthy brain and happy mood! When you heal your gut, you heal from depression.

Probiotic supplements and yogurt contain, at most, a dozen types of bacteria that your gut needs for optimal wellness, but fermented foods, like kimchi and sauerkraut, can provide up to several hundred species of bacteria. For that reason, I highly recommend including ample amounts of these foods into your diet. You can make kimchi yourself, and starter kits are sold at most health food stores. You can also buy ready-made kimchi.

Healthy Oils and Fats

Healthy oils and fats are integral to proper brain function, healthy cell membranes, and for the formation of fats used to make hormones, the latter of which carry messages from glands to cells within your body. Hormones also maintain chemical levels in your bloodstream to help achieve homeostasis or a state of balance within your body. In addition, they play a crucial role in mood regulation, which I will describe in greater detail later in this book.

Healthy oils and fats include: coconut, palm kernel, MCT, almond, walnut, flaxseed, macadamia and olive oils; ghee (clarified butter) and organic butter, as well as nuts, which I noted earlier.

The healthiest oil for cooking is palm kernel oil. This is a fully saturated oil that, when heated, doesn't hydrogenate and form trans fats, or become rancid and oxidize. Coconut and MCT oil are also healthy cooking oils.

Spices

Spices give food an enticing, desirable flavor. Most have anti-oxidant, anti-inflammatory and anti-microbial properties; that is, they fight against pathogenic microbes in the body, and are therefore good for your body and brain, as well as delicious. You can enhance your health and the taste of your foods by preparing foods with a variety of spices. Some spices have specific health benefits. For example, cinnamon can balance blood sugar, and garlic binds heavy metals.

Sea salt is also healthful for most people. The best salt to use is iodized Himalayan salt, which is dug out of the ground in the Himalayan Mountains and originates from a prehistoric seabed. There are no environmental pollutants in this salt like you might find in other salts.

Healthy Sweeteners

Finally, for optimal health, it is crucial to avoid sugar and any artificial sweeteners that cause inflammation and which are toxic to your brain. Aspartame, for instance, has been linked to brain damage in numerous lab studies done on rats,[xxv] and should be avoided as much as sugar, which is inflammatory.

Instead, choose sweeteners made from herbs such as stevia and Chinese monk fruit. These can be used to sweeten beverages, desserts and other foods. They are an excellent alternative to sugar, which is a mood-depressant.

Clean Water and Other Healthy Beverages

Just as it is important to consume clean food, so is it also essential to drink clean water. Unfortunately, just as our food supply has become polluted, so most all tap water nowadays is contaminated by fluoride, chlorine, asbestos, plastics, pesticides, antibiotics, pharmaceutical drugs, heavy metals and other contaminants. Microorganisms, including parasites and viruses, are also prevalent in tap water. Whew, that's quite a list, isn't it?

Most of these toxins can either directly or indirectly influence your mood, and all have damaging effects upon your body when they are present in high enough concentrations. Heavy metals have especially been linked to depression and mood disorders. For instance, a study published in May 2017 in the *The Journal of Clinical Psychiatry* revealed a strong link between cadmium, lead and depression.[xxvi] Similarly, aluminum and mercury have been found to cause depression.

For this reason, it is essential to use a reverse osmosis or carbon block water filter, or bottled water, for all of your drinking, cooking and bathing needs, if you want to avoid contamination by these pollutants. If you don't have a lot of money to spend on water filtration, I recommend at least purchasing a Berkey water filter, which uses a relatively inexpensive carbon block filtration system and is more affordable than some of the higher-tech filtration systems. Some health food stores also sell bottled water that has been purified via reverse osmosis, or you can have purified water delivered to your home in one, three, or five-gallon bottles. Spring water from a reputable source such as Mountain Valley may be best, since it contains life-giving minerals, unlike reverse osmosis water, which does not contain minerals.

For more information, see: MountainValleySpring.com.

If you purchase bottled water, it's preferable to get glass bottles, if you can. Most plastic bottles contain BPA, a chemical that has been linked to hormonal imbalances that can cause depression, especially in women, so this may be an important consideration for some of you.

Finally, I just want to emphasize that there is no such thing as one-size-fits-all when it comes to diet. In my interviews with dozens of doctors, I've found that certain diets seem to work best for some people, while others work better for others. For instance, in recent years, I've been following Steven Gundry, MDs *Plant Paradox* diet, which is a gut-healing diet, the principles of which are somewhat similar to those that I share here, with the difference that Dr. Gundry recommends avoiding all lectin-containing foods.

Lectins are a sticky substance that's found on some plants, and which plants use as part of their defense system, but which damage the human gut. Lectins are found in abundance in grains, legumes, and certain vegetables and fruits, especially those that have small seeds inside. Amazingly, Dr. Gundry and some other doctors I know have found their patients' neurological symptoms to subside significantly when they followed this diet for six months or more. It is a bit challenging to follow at first, but some people have found it to be well worth the effort. To learn more, see: DrGundry.com.

Another gut healing diet that many have found to be beneficial is the Gut and Psychology Syndrome (GAPS) diet. This diet is specifically targeted toward those with autism and other mental disorders, so you may want to give it a try, too. To learn more, see: GapsDiet.com.

In summary, what you eat will powerfully influence your mood and overall health. If you are used to consuming comfort foods such as pasta and cereal, or processed or otherwise unhealthy foods, I realize that it can be very difficult to change your eating habits. I know that it was for me, at first! But I think you'll find that the rewards that you reap by doing so will be more than worth it! Just start with small changes. Don't try to radically change your diet overnight, unless that idea really excites you, but know that by doing one thing at a time, over time, you will be well on your way to a healthier mind and body. Remember, God will help you!

Chapter Ten

Restore Your Brain Chemistry with Nutrition

The Power of Amino Acids to Rebuild Neurotransmitters

As you probably know by now, your brain chemistry is influenced by many factors, including your genes, environmental toxins and infections, nutrient deficiencies, your gut health and trauma. Your beliefs and thoughts also affect your chemistry, but your chemistry also affects your thoughts! That's why, for those of us who battle or have battled depression, there is value in learning to think God's thoughts, but there is also value in supporting and healing your biochemistry so that you are better enabled to think His thoughts! The brain, mind and spirit all work together, so when your brain is compromised, it *can* affect your ability to "take every thought captive." (2 Corinthians 10:5). God's Spirit within you is greater than your chemical imbalances, but the battle in the flesh can be fierce when your chemistry is a mess. So, don't be hard on yourself if you have struggled to "be more positive" or think the right thoughts! You are waging a difficult war.

First of all, it is common for people with depression to have neurotransmitter imbalances. Chronic neurological illness and other conditions deplete neurotransmitters, as do nutritional deficiencies, toxins and prolonged emotional trauma. Because of this, you may find that supporting and balancing your neurotransmitters is incredibly helpful for your recovery.

Neurotransmitters are chemical messengers that coordinate the transmission of signals between nerve cells in your brain and throughout your body. They play a crucial role in your mental, physical and emotional wellbeing, and regulate a multitude of functions including memory, cognition, concentration, alertness, energy, appetite, pain, sleep and of course, the emotions. They affect every cell, organ and system of your body, and are linked to your immune and endocrine (or hormonal) systems. This means that neurotransmitter imbalances can cause a variety of health problems, including depression and anxiety.

In my own battle with depression, I discovered that I had severe dopamine, norepinephrine and serotonin deficiencies, probably caused by a combination of factors: childhood trauma, prolonged illness, a poor diet, and possibly, genetic defects. Serotonin, norepinephrine and dopamine all play a powerful role in mood regulation. In addition, dopamine gives you energy, improves your cognition and mental processing, and, like serotonin, makes you happy. Serotonin is better known for its mood-enhancing effects but it also has other benefits; it reduces pain, helps you sleep, and can give you a sense of peace and inner calm.

If you battle depression, it's worthwhile to get your neurotransmitters tested at a reputable lab to find out whether imbalances in these or other neurotransmitters are contributing to your depression. I use Sabre Sciences in California to do my testing, but there are other good labs out there, the names of which I will share later in this chapter.

Other neurotransmitters affect your mood, but these are primary. If you battle anxiety along with depression—and indeed, the effects of these two conditions often overlap and intertwine—you may also benefit from testing your GABA (or gamma-amino butyric acid) levels. GABA is your body's most important calming neurotransmitter. It helps you to rest and relax and also promotes restful sleep by decreasing neuron firing in your brain.

Later, I will share some powerful amino acids and other supplements that you can take that will help to balance your neurotransmitters. These supplements can reduce or completely eliminate your need to take antidepressants or sedative drugs, especially when you combine them with a healthy diet and the appropriate nutritional co-factors, or supportive nutrients.

Drug companies, through the billions that they spend on ads, have convinced many people in America that they need pharmaceutical remedies to combat depression, or any other malady for that matter. But consider this—you don't have depression because you have a drug deficiency! Your body and brain are lacking nutrients and bio-chemicals that, when replenished, can often completely reverse the problem. Yet pharmaceutical companies have brainwashed many of us into believing that we just have a genetic issue that requires a drug to fix.

Please don't feel badly if you have needed to take drugs to feel okay or to function, though. I know how agonizingly difficult depression can be, and you sometimes just do what you have to do to get by and survive. I took antidepressants and sedatives myself periodically for nearly a decade, to manage Lyme disease symptoms, until God showed me that there was a better way to heal. Weaning off of these drugs was a challenge, but paradoxically, one of the best decisions that I've ever made to regain my health.

If you have been on these types of medications for years, I don't recommend just quitting them "cold turkey," and if you're not ready to get off of them, that's okay, too. Just know that there are many other tools that can help you to recover from depression, and not just manage it, and which don't involve pharmaceutical medication. It may take time to heal your body using these tools, but it can be done.

Also, while anti-depressants and sedatives helped me in the short run to overcome depression and other symptoms of Lyme disease, over the long run, they worsened my symptoms. This is because drugs don't add anything to your body that it needs to heal; in fact, they can actually damage or further deplete your brain chemistry. When I first started taking the medications, I didn't know that there were better options out there.

So again, don't feel badly if you've had to take medicine to get by. The American Medical Association, which is funded by pharmaceutical companies, doesn't teach conventionally trained doctors how to heal the brain (and the rest of the body for that matter) with nutrition. They only teach them how to manage symptoms so many doctors don't even know how to help their patients any other way except with drugs. Later, I share some tips for weaning off of antidepressant and sedative drugs, if you feel led to do so.

Amino Acid Therapy

Amino acids provide the building blocks for neurotransmitters. As I mentioned, serotonin, dopamine and norepinephrine are three of the most important mood regulating neurotransmitters, but they also promote healthy sleep, energy and cognition and can even lessen pain. Other neurotransmitters, like acetylcholine and GABA, have mood enhancing effects, but serotonin, dopamine and norepinephrine are primary.

Tryptophan and 5-HTP are two amino acids that your body uses to make serotonin, which, as I mentioned, is a calming and powerful mood promoting neurotransmitter. You have probably heard about 5-HTP and tryptophan, and perhaps even tried these amino acids, but what you may not know is that they don't always work that well in the body unless the body also has sufficient amounts of certain nutritional co-factors to synthesize or make serotonin from them. Some people also have liver problems or genetic issues that prevent them from properly synthesizing and breaking down neurotransmitters, so if you find that this is true for you, you may not benefit from taking amino acids unless you also have the proper liver-supportive nutrients to make them work in your body.

A surprising number of people actually have these issues; in fact, I had my genes tested and my results revealed that I had what's called a "double mutation" in the genes that play a role in creating and breaking down neurotransmitters. A double mutation is bad news because it means that I inherited genes from both of my parents that potentially compromised my body's ability to properly make and break down neurotransmitters.

Some people who have a double mutation in these genes battle severe psychiatric issues, but the good news is, God is greater than our genes and can override our fleshly DNA with His DNA, according to our faith in Jesus' sacrifice on the Cross. But if you're not there yet, don't worry—because science has also proven that we can influence the expression of our genes by our lifestyle and dietary choices.

A health care practitioner who once analyzed my gene report said, "I've only met one other person who has had a double gene mutation in those same genes as you, and she battled crippling psychiatric issues." I am so thankful that God that He helped me find a way out from my own crippling depression, in spite of my apparently negative genetic profile!

You don't have to be a victim of your genes, either. So don't despair if your whole family battles depression and/or you believe that you have genetic issues that are causing your depression. Your genes don't have to determine your destiny!

Later, I will share some additional nutrients that you can take to help your body to synthesize neurotransmitters from amino acids. You'll want to discuss these with a skilled naturopath or integrative doctor and ideally, get tested to discover which ones you may benefit from. Genetic tests can provide insights into your body's ability to synthesize, utilize and break down neurotransmitters, and can be helpful for determining the nutritional support that you may need. Organic acid tests (OAT) tests do the same, but you'll want to make sure to work with an integrative doctor who knows how to interpret them. The Great Plains Laboratory offers a quality OAT test.

For information, visit: www.greatplainslaboratory.com. Some resources for finding a good doctor are found at the end of this book, in the References section.

If you can't afford genetic or other types of testing, you might ask your doctor to give you a trial treatment of amino acid therapy, to see how you respond. This is less ideal but can sometimes provide enough insight into what supplements you may need. Otherwise, it's best to have your doctor do a complete amino acid and neurotransmitter profile, which are available through many sophisticated labs and compounding pharmacies such as:

- Sabre Sciences (SabreSciences.com)
- NeuroScience (WhyNeuroScience.com)
- Pharmasan (Pharmasan.com)
- BioHealth Diagnostics (BioHealthLab.com)

Some people, especially those who battle other chronic health issues in addition to depression, have commented to me that they feel worse when they take amino acids. I have at times, too. This can be due to several factors. First, and as I just mentioned, your body may not be able to synthesize neurotransmitters from the amino acids, and you may require additional nutrients so that your body will use the amino acids properly.

Secondly, if you are highly deficient in certain amino acids and/or neurotransmitters, you can also feel worse when you first start amino acid therapy. If neurotransmitter testing reveals that you are deficient in certain neurotransmitters and amino acids, you may want to ask your doctor to prescribe you low doses of the appropriate amino acids, and then slowly work your way up on the dosing. Taking a dose that is too high, too soon, can make you feel worse.

The first time that I took a 5-HTP product I actually became more brain fogged, depressed and fatigued. I mistakenly concluded that amino acids were not helpful for me. Unfortunately, I continued to suffer for several years after that, until I realized that the problem wasn't that my body didn't need 5-HTP, but rather, that it couldn't make serotonin from the 5-HTP without a little help. Once I discovered the nutrients that my body needed to synthesize serotonin from 5-HTP, I actually became more energetic, clear-headed, and emotionally balanced after I took these nutrients, in combination with the 5-HTP.

You can purchase 5-HTP, tryptophan and all of the other amino acids that I describe in this chapter at your local health food store or at many online retailers. Quality varies among the products, so it's a good idea to purchase one that has been recommended by a reputable health care practitioner. Personally, I have found the NeuroScience products to be very effective, although they are more expensive than some other amino acid supplements. To learn more about NeuroScience's products, visit the site: NeuroScienceInc.com.

If you take antidepressants or other mood-altering medications, you'll want to first consult with your doctor to see if amino acids are appropriate for you. This is especially important if you are considering 5-HTP or L-tryptophan, as these amino acids are sometimes contraindicated in those who use anti-depressants, as the two remedies together can occasionally cause a condition known as serotonin syndrome. Therefore, if you are taking an antidepressant, use amino acids with caution and only under the guidance of a qualified health care practitioner who understands how to combine medication with amino acids and other nutrients.

Dopamine and norepinephrine are two other important neurotransmitters that powerfully regulate mood. The body makes norepinephrine from dopamine. Therefore, the amino acid precursors to both dopamine and norepinephrine are L-phenylalanine and L-tyrosine. These amino acids can increase your energy, and so are best taken in the morning or early afternoon.

In addition, for best results, serotonin and dopamine should both be balanced in the body. This allows each neurotransmitter to function optimally. One of my former doctors, Jeremy Kaslow, MD, who is an expert in neurotransmitter balancing, taught me this. Both neurotransmitters regulate mood and cognition, but dopamine is an excitatory neurotransmitter that also gives you energy, while serotonin is more calming and promotes sleep at night.

You may find L-tyrosine to be more powerful than L-phenylalanine for producing dopamine in your body because it's one step closer to dopamine on the amino acid synthesis chain so your body doesn't have to do as much work to convert it to the final product. Similarly, 5-HTP may be more powerful than tryptophan because it's one step closer on the amino acid synthesis chain than serotonin.

Therefore, if you are sensitive to supplements, you may want to try L-tryptophan before 5-HTP, and L-phenylalanine before L-tyrosine. However, if you have gene methylation issues that you know make it difficult for your body to make neurotransmitters from amino acids, you may benefit more from L-tyrosine and 5-HTP. Still, some people do best by taking some combination of all four amino acids. For instance, Dr. Kaslow once told me that some of his patients fare best by taking both 5-HTP and tryptophan at bedtime, not just one or the other. Dr. Kaslow has some great articles on neurotransmitter support. You can read these on his site: DrKaslow.com.

The dosages and types of amino acids that you may benefit from will depend on your symptoms and lab test results, so again, it's best to get tested and work with your doctor to find out what you need. A typical regimen may involve starting out with a 50 mg capsule of 5-HTP before bedtime, and then increasing that dose over time until you feel better. Typical doses range from 50 mg up to 300 mg daily.

Similarly, to increase dopamine production (and norepinephrine), a typical regimen may involve taking 100 mg of L-tyrosine daily, and slowly increasing that dose over time until you feel better. Typical L-tyrosine doses range from 100-1,000 mg daily. If you experience anxiety or heart palpitations, you'll want to lower the dose. Again, it is best to work with a naturopath or integrative doctor to determine what you need.

As you take these supplements, monitor your mood, mental function, energy, pain levels, and sleep patterns to see how these change over time. If the supplements are beneficial for you, you should notice positive changes in your symptoms within a few weeks. It's also best to test one amino acid at a time, to see how you respond to each.

Nutritional Co-Factors That Help Your Body to Make and Utilize Neurotransmitters

As I mentioned, amino acids may not work properly in your body if you take the wrong product, dosage or combination of nutrients, or if you need nutritional co-factors, which help your body to synthesize, utilize and break down neurotransmitters. This is important to understand if you have tried amino acids before but not had good results from them.

I have found that many people, especially those who battle chronic neurological diseases and/or have genetic issues that prevent them from effectively synthesizing and breaking down neurotransmitters, need additional nutritional support when taking amino acids. Some common nutrients, or methylators, as they are called, which help the body to synthesize neurotransmitters from amino acids, include:

- SAM-e
- Methyl-folate (a bioavailable form of folate)
- P5P (pyridoxyl phosphate, which is a bioavailable form of Vitamin B-6)
- Vitamin B-12 (the methyl form works best for most people)

In addition, your body needs an adequate supply of zinc, magnesium, vitamin C and vitamin B-6 to make serotonin from 5-HTP, so if you are deficient in these nutrients, taking one or more of these may be helpful. As well, you may want to ask your doctor about trying a low trial dose of one or more of the methylating substances, such as SAM-e, methyl-folate or Vitamin B-12, according to your lab results.

A small dose of SAM-e would be about 50 mg, taken in the morning (as it can disrupt your sleep when taken at night). Again, even if you do lab testing, you may find that you need to experiment with the methylators and co-factor nutrients to find the one(s) that will work best for you, along with the appropriate dosages.

When I first started using supplements, I found that I could not tolerate more than half a capsule of SAMe. If I took more, it actually kept me up at night and caused insomnia, but a small amount helped my body to utilize the amino acids that I needed to get proper rest. I then introduced a small amount of P5P into my regimen, and finally, methylfolate. I added them to my regimen one at a time, so that I could gauge my response to each.

I highly recommend supplementing in this way, following your doctor's recommendations and doing lab tests to determine what your body needs, as taking too much of any one methylator or co-factor nutrient can cause side effects, such as insomnia or excitability. In any case, it is always best to consult with a knowledgeable integrative doctor and/or compounding pharmacist for help in balancing your chemistry.

Finally, GABA, which is a calming amino acid in addition to a neurotransmitter, can be helpful for managing any anxiety that you may have that is linked to the depression. GABA helps you to relax and is a great substitute for sedative drugs, although in some cases may occasionally worsen depression.

GABA is also a fantastic sleep aid. Insomnia is common in people who battle depression and I have found GABA supplements to be one of the most powerful tools for helping me to recover from depression-induced insomnia, and I continue to use it to this day. If you struggle to sleep, you can read more about GABA and other novel sleep solutions in my downloadable E-book:

Beyond a Glass of Milk and a Hot Bath: Advanced Sleep Solutions for People with Chronic Insomnia, which you can find at: ConnieStrasheim.org.

My favorite GABA product is Kavinace, which is made by Neuro Science. Kavinace is a bioavailable form of GABA, and an especially great product for those of you who don't respond well to pure GABA and/or have genetic defects that prevent your body from effectively utilizing amino acids. Kavinace costs more than just plain ol' GABA but can make a world of difference in your wellbeing. If you haven't tried Kavinace, I encourage you ask your doctor about it, especially if neurotransmitter testing indicates that you need GABA. It is a very powerful natural sleep aid.

You can purchase Kavinace at many online retailers such as: PureFormulas.com, or at the NeuroScience website: NeuroScienceInc.com, although you will need a doctor's order if you purchase products from the company's website.

The Role of Other Neurotransmitters in Mood Regulation

Other neurotransmitters play a role in mood regulation, but those that I just described to you are among the most powerful. Acetylcholine is another neurotransmitter that has a positive effect upon mood, although its impact is generally less significant than that of serotonin and dopamine. However, it can greatly improve cognition and mental function, which are often compromised in people who battle depression.

I've found that taking choline, which is a precursor that the body uses to make acetylcholine, has also been very helpful for improving my mood and reducing other symptoms of depression, like brain fog, slow mental processing, indecision, and memory loss. All of the body's cell membranes are partially comprised of choline, so by taking choline, either orally, trans- dermally or even intravenously, you can also help to heal all of your cells. By healing cell membranes, choline also helps to detoxify the cells, which can also, as a side effect, mitigate depression.

Finally, taurine is an amino acid that is found in high levels in the central nervous system, and which helps to modulate and promote healthy levels of GABA, as well as a neurotransmitter called glutamate. Glutamate is an excitatory neurotransmitter that plays a crucial role in mental function but which is found in excess in many people, especially those with neurodegenerative diseases and depression. Excessively high levels of glutamate can cause inflammation and depression, so if your testing shows that you have high glutamate due to disease or toxicity, you may benefit from taurine supplements.

Another benefit of taurine is that studies have shown it to help prevent neuron damage caused by excessive levels of glutamate.[xxvii] Taurine can be purchased at many online retailers and at health food stores.

How to Determine Whether Amino Acid Therapy Is Right for You

In the end, the steps that you'll want to take to determine whether amino acid therapy is right for you, include:

1) Doing a complete amino acid and neurotransmitter profile through a reputable lab such as Sabre Sciences, NeuroScience, and/or BioHealth Diagnostics.
For more information, visit the websites:
SabreSciences.com, NeuroScienceInc.com, and
BiohealthLab.com, respectively.

2) Doing a trial treatment of amino acid therapy. I always recommend working with a doctor on this, so that he or she can help you determine an appropriate supplement regimen and adjust it if needed.

3) Supplementing with the appropriate co-factors that aid in neurotransmitter synthesis, such as zinc, magnesium and vitamin C, the levels of which are depleted in many of us, due to our nutrient-deficient food supply.

4) Supplementing with methylators, or nutritional co-factors that help your body to make neurotransmitters from amino acids. Take these only if your test results indicate that you need nutritional or methylation support, you respond poorly to amino acids, and/or your doctor tells you that you need them.

Clues that you may have a genetic defect that is compromising your body's ability to utilize amino acids include:

1) Having a negative reaction to amino acids
2) Genetic test results that indicate you need methylation support
3) Test results that indicate that you have an amino acid deficiency, but taking the appropriate amino acids seems to produce no change in your wellbeing.

The most commonly used methylators or nutrients that aid in neurotransmitter synthesis include:

- SAM-e
- Vitamins B-6 (or pyridoxyl phosphate, P5P)
- Vitamin B-12 (methyl B-12 tends to be the most effective form of this B vitamin for most people). You may need one or more of these
- Methyl-folate

*Tips for Weaning off of Anti-Depressant and
Sedative Drugs*

As I mentioned earlier, I periodically used sedative drugs and anti-depressants for nearly a decade. My doctors prescribed them to help me sleep, as well as for the depression. They helped me in the short term, but after a while, they quit working and worsened my symptoms.

Because of this, I determined to find a better solution for my sleep, mood and other related symptoms, and so I slowly tapered off of the medications that I was on, one at a time. These included the anti-depressant amitriptyline and a sedative drug called lorazepam. What finally convinced me to let them both go was when I realized that lorazepam was affecting my memory, and ability to reason and function cognitively. Benzodiazepines are one of the most addictive types of drugs there are, so I won't lie—letting go of it was hard. But with God's help, I did!

The weaning process took many months, and I battled many withdrawal symptoms such as severe insomnia (paradoxically, one of the conditions that the drug was intended to treat!), anxiety, chest pain, severe depression, heart palpitations, back pain, fatigue, hallucinations, mild seizures, shakiness, and more. However, had I known then what I know now about how to restore the brain and body during and after benzodiazepine and antidepressant use, I think the withdrawal process would have been much easier.

If you are addicted to antidepressants, sedatives and/or other sleep medications but want a better solution to manage your symptoms, I want to encourage you that it *is* possible to get off of these medications and heal your brain with nutrition and other tools. However, it is *imperative* to work with a competent doctor or other health care practitioner who understands nutrition, drug addiction and how to heal and restore the body's chemistry with nutrition. In this chapter I'll give you a basic roadmap of tools, so that you have an idea about where to start. You can then begin to seek out the resources that you'll need to begin the process.

Of course, some of you who are reading this may need to continue on your medications for a period of time, or even indefinitely, to manage your symptoms. But know this—all drugs have side effects, and there are often better ways to manage depression over the long term. Not always, but often.

If you are thinking, *but you don't understand how I feel*! Or, *I have a genetic issue that requires me to take these drugs* –that may be true, and your doctor may recommend that you stay on your medication. I'm just saying that there are often better ways to heal and/or manage symptoms. God showed me a better way. And if I can do it, I believe that with His help, you can, too!

Again though, drug withdrawal can be difficult, and is definitely not a do-it-yourself endeavor. You need God to help you, as well as the support of at least one good friend and/or professional counselor, in addition to a doctor, and that doesn't mean a psychiatrist who tells you to taper off of your meds in just two weeks, or even a month.

If you've been on antidepressants or sedative drugs for more than a short period of time, which may be defined as anywhere from 3-6 months to years, it could take you many months to wean off of them, depending on your biochemistry. If you have been on these medications for just a few months, you may be able to wean off of them in just a matter of weeks, but if it has been longer than that; say, six months or more, you may need months, if not a year or more to wean off of them completely. Do not rush the process. I can't overemphasize how important that is. Going too fast can cause relapses and dangerous, even life-threatening drug withdrawal symptoms, so please do not do it on your own, without medical and professional guidance.

It took me two years to fully wean off of the antidepressant and benzodiazepine medications that I was on, and perhaps several more years to really heal my brain and the rest of my body from the effects of those medications (and I may still be healing, in fact). But again, I believe that I can help to shorten the runway for you by sharing with you some of the tools that I discovered to be helpful for my healing, both during and after the weaning process. Feel free to discuss any the following with your doctor, if he or she is open-minded about natural medicine, and then research them in greater depth on your own.

1). Amino acid therapy, especially GABA, 5-HTP and L-tyrosine. These amino acids were a powerful part of my supplement toolkit and took the place of the antidepressants and sedative that I was addicted to.

Sedatives, or benzodiazepines, act as a potent type of artificial GABA in the body, so taking supplemental GABA can help to make the transition off of these kinds of drugs a bit easier. Five-HTP and L-tyrosine may alleviate depression, fatigue, insomnia, pain and other symptoms commonly caused by drug withdrawal, and over the long run can often replace the need for anti-depressant therapy.

2). Brain wave entrainment. This therapy sends energetic frequencies from a neurofeedback device to your brain, to measure your brain waves. It then utilizes that information to create a customized frequency signal, which it feeds back to your brain via sound and light waves. The signal has the effect of modulating your brain waves.

I have found the entrainment therapy devices from a company called Clear Mind to be especially useful for treating rebound insomnia and other symptoms that occur as a part of sedative and antidepressant medication withdrawal. To learn more about brain wave entrainment therapy, see: ClearMindCenter.com. The brain wave entrainment devices are also useful for healing the brain from depression and other neurological disorders.

Less expensive devices are also sold at ToolsforWellness.com, although I have no experience with this company's products so I can't attest to their effectiveness. To learn more about brain wave entrainment, see Dr. Cowden's and my 2014 book: *BioEnergetic Tools for Wellness.*

Many clinics do brain wave entrainment sessions, as well. To find one in your area, you can do an Internet search by inputting the term "neurofeedback clinics," along with your city and state, into the search engine.

3). Nutritional support. The better your diet is, the lesser will be the effects of any drug withdrawal symptoms that you experience. I highly recommend a diet that follows the guidelines that I shared in this book, or read Dr. Cowden's and my 2014 book, *Foods that Fit a Unique You* for more information on a healthy, anti-inflammatory diet that can be tailored to your specific needs.

4). Prayer. God can heal you or sustain you supernaturally, and/or enable you to do above and beyond anything that you can do on your own in the natural realm. I have a friend who was supernaturally healed of drug addiction and required no other tools to get well. God can do this for you as well, or He may supernaturally anoint tools in the natural realm that He wants to use to heal you. Regardless, He will help you to heal and get off of your medication, no matter what method you choose to get well.

In addition, consider joining a faith-based community and enlisting the help of at least several prayer partners as you go through the drug withdrawal process. It will make all the difference in the world. In the meantime, be encouraged and feed your faith by meditating on Jesus' work on the Cross and thanking Him for accelerated and divine healing. Speak healing Scriptures over yourself daily. Doing these things can expedite your recovery.

5). Emotional support. You'll need at least one friend or prayer partner that you can call at any hour of the day, if and when you go through difficult withdrawal symptoms. I was grateful to be able to awaken Bill at 2 or 3 AM whenever the insomnia, depression and/or other symptoms from drug withdrawal became difficult. Bill often encouraged, consoled and prayed for me during those times, which enabled me to endure and keep on going with the process. Support groups can also be helpful.

6). Schedule regular visits with a knowledgeable medical doctor and/or addictions counselor, who can help you to determine how quickly you should taper off of your medications and can monitor you as you go through the process. If you see a conventional doctor or counselor who tells you that you can easily taper off your medications within a week or a month, even though you've been on them for many months or years—run! Many doctors are misinformed about the challenges of drug withdrawal and how long the body needs to re-adjust, even from anti-depressant use, so make sure that you find someone who truly understands the challenges. Again, not everyone will have difficulty getting off of these medications, but some people require many months to taper off of them.

7). Spend time in the sunshine daily and make sure that you nurture your soul and spirit. Do something daily that brings you joy, such as hanging out with God, watching an uplifting television program, reading a good novel, walking in nature, or having coffee with friends.

8). Exercise. This will help your body to heal on multiple levels and stimulate the release of mood-enhancing chemicals called endorphins. I have found walking in nature to be particularly therapeutic for me.

This information is only meant to be a starting point, to give you a broad idea about the tools that are needed to effectively withdraw and heal from the effects of antidepressant and sedative medication addiction. Sometimes, an arsenal of tools is required, but it is possible to get off of these drugs, especially with God's help! And if you aren't ready to take that step right now, or don't feel led to do so, that's okay. Be led by God in your decision-making and listen to what He tells you to do. Only He knows what you need right now.

For more information on how to withdraw from benzodiazepines, I highly recommend the book, *Recovery and Renewal: Your Essential Guide to Overcoming*

Dependency and Withdrawal from Sleeping Pills, Other 'Benzo' Tranquillisers and Antidepressants by addictions counselor Baylissa Frederick. Dr. Frederick also does personal Skype consultations. For more information, visit: recovery-road.org/consultations.

Chapter Eleven

Balance Your Hormones for a Better You

Hormone Imbalances: A Common Cause of Depression

Another common physiological cause of depression, especially in women, is hormonal imbalances. Few things can impact a woman's emotions, mind and body as much as when her hormones are in disarray. Hormonal imbalances are caused by many things, including environmental toxins, illness, stress, trauma, a poor diet and simply, aging.

Consequently, hormonal imbalances are very common in today's toxic world, even among younger men and women. For instance, environmental toxins such as BPA and phthalates (which are chemicals found in plastics), mimic estrogen in the body and cause imbalances of progesterone and estrogen. An excess or deficiency of either hormone can cause depression.

In addition, many of us battle adrenal gland and thyroid dysfunction, both of which can cause depression. The adrenal glands produce hormones such as cortisol, pregnenolone, progesterone, estrogen, and testosterone, all of which have an effect upon the mood, either directly or indirectly (as well as the entire functioning of the body!), as do thyroid hormones. Adrenal and thyroid dysfunction is due to environmental toxins, chronic infections and perhaps most importantly, stress resulting from things like chronic abuse, living a hectic lifestyle, maintaining a poor diet, and living in "fight or flight" mode.

Your adrenal glands are responsible for producing hormones in response to stress, but when there is a constant drain on your body from stress, inflammation, environmental toxicity and other factors, over time, the adrenals can burn out, resulting in a condition that is now widely known as "adrenal fatigue." This results in an underproduction or overproduction of adrenal hormones, especially cortisol. Two major symptoms of adrenal dysfunction are anxiety and depression, in addition to other symptoms like fatigue and insomnia.

When your adrenals malfunction, your thyroid gland will tend to stop functioning properly, as well. This is because your cells require cortisol to uptake and utilize thyroid hormone, so if you have an insufficient amount of cortisol, your thyroid hormones can't do their job. In addition, environmental contaminants such as fluoride are widely known to damage the thyroid. For this and other reasons, adrenal fatigue and adrenal hormone imbalances often lead to thyroid hormone imbalances and vice versa.

Because I spent most of my life living in fear, or "fight-or-flight" mode, I suspect that my adrenal glands and thyroid began to malfunction early on in my life. Lyme disease then caused my hormones to become significantly imbalanced. Because both the thyroid and adrenals affect many processes, another step in my healing journey involved restoring hormonal balance to my body.

You may find that you need to do the same, especially if you battle a chronic health condition in addition to depression or are a woman over the age of 35 and are either pre-menopausal, menopausal or post-menopausal.

You may know that balancing the hormones can be challenging, and I have found that few health care practitioners really know how to do it well, especially for people who have battled serious chronic neurological or autoimmune-like illnesses. The good news is that if you are addressing all of the other factors that are causing the depression, you don't necessarily have to have perfect hormonal balance.

It is beyond the scope of this book to describe in detail every strategy for balancing the hormones, or the endocrine system, because this is a complex subject. For this reason, I will only share with you here, in a very summarized fashion, a few of the most powerful tools that I have found for restoring proper hormonal balance, to provide you with a starting point and food for thought as you pursue further research or consult with an integrative or naturopathic doctor in this area. I especially encourage you to consider hormonal imbalances as a major factor that could be causing or contributing to your depression if you are a woman in your mid-late 30s or older, or if you battle other chronic health conditions in addition to depression.

How to Discover Whether Your Hormones Need Help

First, I recommend asking your doctor to do urine, blood and/or saliva tests to measure your adrenal and thyroid hormone levels. If you don't have a good integrative or naturopathic doctor, you'll want to find one, as many conventional medical doctors, even endocrinologists (yep, you heard right), don't know how to properly balance the hormones. This is because most use outdated, useless tests that tell you little to nothing about how your endocrine, or hormonal system is functioning. They also tend to prescribe synthetic medications that have been recommended or sold to them by pharmaceutical companies, rather than natural bio-identical hormones, which are safer and more compatible with the body.

To find a good integrative and/or holistic doctor, I recommend consulting integrative medical associations such as the Academy for Comprehensive Integrative Medicine (ACIM), the American College for Advancement in Medicine (ACAM), or The Institute for Functional Medicine, for doctor recommendations in your state.

For more information, see: ACIMConnect.com, ACAM.org and/or FunctionalMedicine.org.

Doing research online can also be beneficial. For instance, you could input the terms "Integrative, functional or naturopathic bio-identical hormone doctor (city, state)" into your computer's Internet search engine, and see what you come up with. As part of your research, read online reviews, and learn whatever you can about the practitioner's competency in hormone balancing, because this is a complex area of medicine.

Hormone balancing isn't a do-it-yourself endeavor in any case, so it's important to work with someone who can interpret test results for you and provide appropriate guidance about what you'll need. For your thyroid test, you'll want to do a complete blood panel that measures TSH, T4, T3, Free T3, T3 uptake, Hashimoto's antibodies and perhaps even Reverse T3. The best test for measuring adrenal function is a 24-hour circadian profile, which is a saliva test. You can do this test from home and mail it in to the lab.

For more information on what each of these tests measures and how to support the thyroid, I recommend reading Dr. Datis Kharrazian's book:

Why Do I Still Have Thyroid Symptoms? When My Lab Tests Are Normal: a Revolutionary Breakthrough in Understanding Hashimoto's Disease and Hypothyroidism.

In addition to doing a 24-hour saliva test for your adrenals, and a blood test for your thyroid, your doctor should also evaluate your symptoms to determine whether hormonal imbalances are playing a role in the depression.

This is because all tests have their limitations and none reveals perfectly what's going on in your body. I have known people to occasionally have near normal cortisol levels on a saliva test and yet battle adrenal fatigue, so it's important to work with a doctor who understands endocrine disorders. Ironically, and as I mentioned this is not always (or even usually) a traditional endocrinologist. I, and many others I know have had better results consulting with integrative medical doctors or naturopaths in this area. Such doctors are usually able to diagnose you based on your symptoms, not just test results.

Some of the most common symptoms of adrenal fatigue include:

- Fatigue, especially in the morning
- Post-exertion malaise (which means that you become excessively tired or have an increase in symptoms as a result of doing too much)
- Low blood pressure
- Hypoglycemia, or blood sugar imbalances
- Depression
- Anxiety
- Brain fog
- Gastrointestinal disturbances, especially low stomach acid
- Insomnia
- Weight gain or weight loss
- Orthostatic hypotension, or difficulty standing
- Feeling easily overwhelmed
- Low stamina and an inability to exercise
- Strong cravings for salt and/or sugar

Hypothyroidism, which is the most common thyroid disorder, also causes depression, brain fog, fatigue and insomnia (among other symptoms) but for different reasons. Unfortunately, due to environmental pollution, many people today battle some degree of adrenal fatigue and thyroid dysfunction, even younger adults and those who haven't been diagnosed with a chronic illness.

For an excellent in-depth look at adrenal health, I highly recommend reading adrenal expert Michael Lam, MDs book, *Adrenal Fatigue:Reclaim Your Energy and Vitality with Clinically Proven Natural Programs.*

Tools for Restoring Optimal Adrenal Function

The most crucial step for restoring your adrenal glands and hormonal balance, which may also be the most challenging, yet the least expensive, is to cut down on the stress in your life! If you notice that you are constantly in "fight-or-flight" mode, rushing around, living in fear, taking on too many obligations, living in unhealthy relationships or working a stressful job, I encourage you to ask God to help you reduce that stress.

I realize that this can be difficult if you are living with heavy or multiple challenges, such as a chronic illness, financial hardship, or an abusive relationship, but the truth is, we can all do things to manage our response to challenging situations. This is a foremost step for recovery from this condition. Ask Holy Spirit to help you. A good verse to meditate on to assist you with this might be, "And my God will liberally supply (fill until full) your every need according to His riches in glory in Christ Jesus" (Philippians 4:19).

Next, eliminate all inflammatory foods from your diet, as these foods stress the adrenal glands and cause them to overproduce cortisol, your body's principal stress hormone, which, when released in excess, can keep you awake at night. Common inflammatory foods include: most dairy products, soy, wheat, gluten-containing foods, sugar, and of course, all foods that are excessively processed and which contain artificial ingredients (read: things that you can't grow or find in nature!).

Then, ask your doctor about nutrients and supplements that support adrenal and thyroid function. Some of the most effective for promoting adrenal health and which I have found to be safe for most people, include:

- Vitamin C (anywhere from 1,000-20,000 mg daily, depending on your body's need). Start by taking 1,000 mg per day and adding 500 mg daily, until you reach bowel tolerance. When your stools become slightly loose, reduce the dose slightly. This will be your optimal daily dose. At times during my recovery from Lyme disease, I have needed up to 20 grams (or 20,000 mg) daily of Vitamin C, so don't be surprised if you end up having to take a bit more than you think! By the way, the US RDA's recommendations for Vitamin C are extremely low and insufficient to maintain health. Most of us need much more; an average dose for a healthy person might be 2-5 grams daily. A chronically ill person may need dosages of anywhere from 5-20 grams daily, or even more than that.

- Pantothenic acid or pantethine, also known as Vitamin B5. The adrenal glands love this nutrient! If you have adrenal fatigue, consider including 500 mg or more in your daily regimen.

- Siberian ginseng, ashwagandha and rhodiola. These herbs are adaptogens that help to balance the adrenals and many people seem to tolerate them well.

- Licorice root. Licorice is an excellent remedy if your cortisol levels are too low, since licorice causes your body to retain cortisol so that it stays in your system longer. Long- term use of licorice may cause hypokalemia (or potassium depletion), so you'll want to monitor your potassium levels if you take licorice root long-term. Licorice root also boosts blood pressure, which is a great benefit for those of you who have low blood pressure, which is common in adrenal fatigue. However, it should be used only under physician supervision if you have heart disease, high blood pressure and/or high cortisol levels.

If you have advanced adrenal fatigue, which is characterized by profound fatigue, especially in the morning; anxiety, depression, brain fog, an inability to exercise, weight fluctuations, gastrointestinal disturbances and low morning cortisol levels, or inverted or low cortisol levels across the board on a saliva test, you may also need to take bio-identical hormones and/or adrenal glandular formulas to balance your adrenal hormones. Bio-identical hormones compensate for whatever hormones your adrenal glands may not be making in sufficient amounts and should be prescribed by a doctor who is an expert in bio-identical hormone supplementation.

Some people are averse to taking hormones, and I believe that the decision to take bio-identical hormones should not be taken lightly. At the same time, hormones are not the same as drugs. They are more like nutrients in that they simply make up for what your body is not making. If you are under 35 and you have hormone imbalances, it's worthwhile to see a naturopathic or integrative medical doctor and have him or her test and treat you for underlying causes of hormone imbalances, such as environmental toxins or chronic infections, before you consider hormone replacement therapy.

If you have already tried many natural remedies for adrenal exhaustion and/or you are over 35 years old, you may find supplemental bio-identical hormones such as pregnenolone, progesterone, DHEA, 7-keto DHEA, testosterone and/or (as a last resort) hydrocortisone, to be appropriate treatments for adrenal fatigue. These hormones provide powerful support to the adrenal glands and can help them to recover, while providing your body with the supplemental hormones that it needs in the meantime. The specific hormones that you'll need will depend upon your lab test results and symptoms.

Some of these hormones are more powerful than others, and have profound effects upon the body, so again, you'll want to work with a doctor who thoroughly understands bio-identical hormone replacement when deciding upon which one(s) may be most beneficial for you. It is beyond the scope of this book to describe the function of each of these hormones, so you'll want to do further research on your own to learn about how each of these hormones supports the body. I have found that adequate levels of cortisol and proper estrogen-progesterone balance are especially important for mitigating depression and anxiety in women.

Adrenal glandular formulas, such as those made by Standard Process and Biotics Research (such as Adrenal Dessicated and ADB5 Plus, respectively) contain bovine adrenal gland tissue and other nutrients and are two glandular formulas that are widely recommended by many holistic and integrative doctors to support healthy adrenal function, as well. Ideally, these should also be used under physician supervision, because they may contain active adrenal hormones, and as such, their effects upon the body can be profound. They are also generally used as a last resort to treat adrenal dysfunction when lifestyle changes, nutrition and herbs aren't enough.

For more information see: StandardProcess.com and BioticsResearch.com.

Finally, I have found that brain retraining programs, such as Dynamic Neural Retraining and Ashok Gupta's Amygdala Retraining, can help to heal the adrenals by resetting and restoring the limbic system. This is because when the limbic system gets stuck in "fight or flight" mode, it triggers the adrenal glands to constantly release stress hormones, which in turn burns them out and fatigues the body.

For more information on these training programs, visit: RetrainingTheBrain.com and LimbicRetraining.com.

Tools for Restoring Thyroid Function

Hypothyroidism is a condition in which the thyroid gland fails to produce adequate levels of hormones, or the cells can't uptake and utilize those hormones. It is common in our toxic world and has been shown to disrupt serotonin signaling in the brain. This means that the brain requires sufficient thyroid hormones to function properly, so having low thyroid function can contribute to depression and degeneration in the brain.

Hashimoto's thyroiditis, an autoimmune thyroid disease, can cause the metabolism to be either overly active or overly depressed. When this happens, the person experiences mood swings that can mimic the symptoms of bipolar disorder and cause some people to be misdiagnosed as bipolar. So if you battle bi-polar depression and have never had your thyroid checked, you may find it worthwhile to get a test for autoimmune thyroiditis.

If you battle mild hypothyroidism, you may find that supporting your thyroid with thyroid hormone precursors such as iodine, selenium and L-tyrosine, which your body uses to make thyroid hormone, will restore your thyroid function back to normal. However, you'll want to work with your doctor to determine the specific products and doses that you'll need.

Alternatively, and if your thyroid dysfunction is more severe, as indicated by your symptoms and thyroid lab test results, you may benefit from taking supplemental bio-identical thyroid hormone. If you have severe adrenal fatigue along with thyroid dysfunction, you may respond better to a prescription of pure bio-identical T3 hormone, which is the active form of thyroid hormone that your body uses, rather than a combination of T4/T3 or pure T4. This is because in people with severe adrenal fatigue or autoimmune disease, the body will often make Reverse T3 from T4 hormone (which is an inactive form of thyroid hormone) instead of the active T3 hormone that the body needs, and which counteracts the effects of T3.

To learn more about the interaction between adrenal and thyroid hormones, I recommend reading Dr. Lam's book, *Adrenal Fatigue - Reclaim Your Energy and Vitality with Clinically Proven Natural Programs* as well as Janie Bowthorpe's book, *Stop the Thyroid Madness*. If you're not a scholar or feel overwhelmed by the idea of learning about a bunch of medical concepts, at least find an integrative or functional medicine doctor to help you with this aspect of your recovery. These doctors will treat the root causes of disease, rather than just symptoms, which is why it is so important to find a good one. Trust me, it's worth the search, the time and money to find the right help!

Balancing Your Hormones After Age 35

If you are a pre-menopausal or menopausal woman, you may find that your sleep, mood and energy have become less than ideal, or even downright awful in recent years. Indeed, many women between the ages of 35-45, start experiencing symptoms of depression, insomnia, fatigue, and brain fog, among others—a few days or even a week or two before their menstrual cycles begin, as the hormones estrogen and progesterone start to become imbalanced as a natural result of aging.

Many women in midlife also develop an imbalance of progesterone and estrogen partly because, as I mentioned earlier, many environmental toxins act like estrogens in the body, and cause a condition called estrogen dominance, which is linked to depression. Phthalates, which are chemicals that are found in plastics, are a particular type of toxin that artificially elevates estrogen in the body, and we are all filled with these chemicals.

Conversely, low estrogen, which many women experience during and after menopause can cause depression since studies show that healthy, natural estrogen (not the xenoestrogens produced by toxins) increases serotonin in the brain.

Testosterone deficiency has been linked to depression in men, since testosterone plays a crucial role in brain function, including mood regulation. Studies have confirmed that men are more likely to be depressed if their testosterone levels are low.

Replacing the hormones that your body is missing or balancing them with natural remedies such as herbs and bio-identical hormones can be a crucial and incredibly valuable step to mitigating depression caused by hormonal imbalances. For instance, if you are a pre-menopausal woman, transdermal progesterone crème, which is available at most health food and online stores, can help to balance the ratio of progesterone to estrogen in your body during the second half of your menstrual cycle. It can also mitigate depression caused by imbalances of estrogen and progesterone, which are common in women over 35. Taking 5-HTP or another serotonin precursor can also be helpful.

If you are menopausal or post-menopausal, you may also need to supplement with bio-identical estrogen. Like all hormone replacement therapy, you shouldn't just take progesterone or estrogen willy-nilly though, as they have profound effects upon your body, for better or for worse. Do a lab test to determine whether you need these, or any other hormone.

In addition, some supplements can help to remove or block the effects of unwanted xenoestrogens, or chemicals in the environment that mimic estrogen in the body. DIM, or di-indolylmethane, may be one of the most famous of these. Certain foods such as flax seeds and sprouts, and cruciferous vegetables such as broccoli, cauliflower and cabbage are rich in indole-3-carbinol (I3C), a compound that the body converts to diindolylmethane (DIM). DIM supplements can also be purchased online. They too, can be very powerful.

A friend of mine who had a large ovarian cyst was able to avoid surgery to remove the cyst simply by taking high doses (about 300 mg) of DIM daily. This is because ovarian cysts have been linked to estrogen dominance, and DIM helps to clear estrogen from the body.

According to gynecologist Christiane Northrup MD, author of *Women's Bodies, Women's Wisdom*, high estrogen levels in pre-menopausal women are also associated with deficiencies of the vitamin B complex, especially vitamins B6 and B12, as well as vitamins C and E, magnesium and selenium. The liver requires adequate amounts of these nutrients to break down and inactivate estrogen, so you may want to also consider supplementing your diet with these vitamins and minerals, if you battle PMS or pre-menopausal symptoms that include depression and/or your test results indicate that you need them.

I began taking bio-identical hormones in the form of transdermal creams around age 37. My repertoire included pregnenolone, 7-keto DHEA and progesterone, all of which support the adrenal glands and proper production of a variety of hormones. When I began taking these hormones, my energy, mood and mental function all improved dramatically.

I actually wish that I had started taking bio-identical hormones sooner, since my hormone levels had been low for years; probably due to a combination of stress and illness, and I was exhausted, brain fogged, depressed and continually sleep-deprived. I also discovered in my late 30s that I was extremely deficient in healthy HDL cholesterol. The body creates brain tissue and hormones from cholesterol, so this meant that my body didn't have enough raw materials to make all of the hormones that I needed in the first place. And if you don't have the raw material, or building blocks to make hormones, then nothing in your body will work right.

Low cholesterol is just as dangerous as high cholesterol, so it's important to check your cholesterol as part of your wellness protocol. This is especially important if you have another chronic health condition. If you have low levels of healthy, or HDL cholesterol, you'll want to find ways to increase your levels of this crucial lipid. Cod fish liver oil, duck eggs and caviar are three of the most cholesterol rich foods, so you may find that supplementing with these is helpful, if your cholesterol is low.

According to one of my doctor friends, low cholesterol has also been linked to poor liver function and blocked bile ducts. Therefore, doing a liver cleanse may be helpful for restoring cholesterol levels. Incidentally, a clogged or toxic liver can also affect your mood, so doing a cleanse may be a good idea, anyway! For more information on a good liver cleanse to try, ask your doctor or a trusted healthcare practitioner. Some liver cleanses can be a little intense, so you'll want to do one that's appropriate for your current level of health.

In Summary

Depression can be caused by hormonal imbalances, especially in women over 35 or people with other chronic health challenges. Adrenal fatigue, hypothyroidism and other thyroid conditions, as well as hormonal changes after age 35, are some of the most common hormonal triggers for depression. Imbalances can powerfully influence your mood and recovery, so I recommend getting your hormones tested, especially if you are a woman or man over age 35 or are battling a chronic illness.

I believe that you'll be excited once you see the tremendous benefits that can result when you balance your hormones with the proper nutrients, bio-identical hormones and a healthy diet. Indeed, addressing this aspect of your health can go a long way toward improving your mood and quality of life.

Supporting my adrenal glands and thyroid with nutrition and bio-identical hormone replacement was only one piece of the depression puzzle for me, but it was one of the most important. That said, you might find that you don't need as many or even the same tools that I did. In fact, chances are, you won't, unless you are also battling a half-dozen major health issues that are profoundly affecting your mind and body. I'm just covering as many bases as possible here, in the hopes that you will find some tools that will work for you.

Finally, I encourage you to speak healing Scriptures or words of divine healing over your hormones daily, so that you don't have to take hormones forever, or perhaps even at all. This goes for any other biochemical imbalances that you have, and any other treatments that you do. By doing this, you can cause your natural treatments to become supernatural, which can in turn expedite your healing!

Chapter Twelve

Resolve Other Biochemical Causes of Depression

It used to be that neurotransmitter and hormonal imbalances were viewed by the medical community as the main physiological causes of depression, but research shows that other phenomena, such as inflammation, insulin resistance, nutritional deficiencies, mitochondrial dysfunction, and oxidative stress may also cause or contribute to depression. In addition, chronic infections are a major, yet largely unrecognized cause of depression. In this chapter, I will share with you on a basic level, how and why all of these factors can cause depression and what you can do to heal your body and brain from their effects. Again, each of these subjects is complex and entire books could be written about each one, so you'll want to just use the information here as a starting point to do further research on your own, or to share with your doctors.

Balance Your Body's Micronutrients

Dietary micronutrients, including vitamins, minerals and essential fatty acids, affect your brain and nervous system function, in addition to the amino acids and neurotransmitter co-factors that I discussed earlier. For this reason, you may find it useful to do a vitamin, fatty acid and mineral profile test, to evaluate your cellular level of micronutrients and make sure that your brain and the rest of your body have what they need to function properly. Spectra Cell Laboratories is one lab that does this type of testing. For more information, see: SpectraCell.com.

B-complex vitamins, which are used as co-factors by your body to produce neurotransmitters, are among the most important nutrients that support nervous system health. I already mentioned Vitamins B-12 and B-6, but adequate levels of niacin and folate are also important.

Vitamin D is another nutrient that's critical for brain and nervous system health. Many North Americans are highly deficient in Vitamin D, because they don't spend enough time in the sunshine. Vitamin D acts more like a hormone than a vitamin in the body and plays a crucial role in mood and immune system regulation. Vitamin D deficiencies have been found in people with Seasonal Affective Disorder (or SAD), a type of depression caused by a lack of exposure to sunlight during the winter months.

Because Vitamin D plays a vital role in supporting mood and overall health, it's a good idea to get your Vitamin D levels tested and take a Vitamin D-3 supplement, if needed. Most integrative doctors consider a normal range of Vitamin D to be above 60 mg/dl. According to integrative doctor Joe Mercola, MD, in his article, "How to Get Your Vitamin D Within to Healthy Ranges" it used to be that the recommended level of Vitamin D was between 40 to 60 nanograms per milliliter (ng/ml). Yet in recent years, the optimal range has been raised to 50-70 ng/ml, and if you are treating cancer or heart disease, it is as high as 70-100 ng/ml.[xxviii]

It's also crucial to have a proper balance of omega-3 to omega-6 essential fatty acids (EFAs) in your body, which come from fatty foods such as healthy cooking oils, nuts, seeds and fish. Fatty acids are important components of nerve cell membranes and play a vital role in neuronal communication. Fatty acid imbalances can impair nerve transmission between nerve cells, leading to cognitive problems and mood issues, including depression.

In a healthy diet, omega-6 EFAs primarily come from cooking oils and nuts, while the best omega-3 EFAs come from high quality fish oils. You need both types of EFAs, but most of us have too much omega-6, which means that we could benefit more from taking some omega-3 EFAs from fish oil to balance things out. Omega-3 essential fatty acids are also highly anti-inflammatory and can mitigate depression caused by inflammation (more on this in the next section). Taking a high-quality fish oil supplement that has been tested to be free of heavy metals is the best way to do that. Choose a supplement that has studies backing its effectiveness and which confirm its purity. Nordic Naturals is one company that has a good reputation for effectiveness and purity. For more information, see: NordicNaturals.com.

Cut Down on Oxidative Stress, Inflammation and Histamine, Three Major Causes of Depression

Oxidative Stress (OS) is a general term that's used to describe damage that occurs to your cells when your body's ability to remove free radicals (which are byproducts of toxicity and metabolism) via its antioxidant system, fail to keep up with the amount of free radicals in your body. When there are too many free radicals in your body, it can't cope and the result is inflammation and cellular damage. Nowadays, most of us have high amounts of oxidative stress, due mostly to environmental toxicity, stress and our hectic lifestyles. The resultant inflammation and cellular damage can cause or contribute to depression and other brain and nervous system disorders.

Therefore, you may find that reducing oxidative stress and inflammation can help to mitigate your symptoms, especially if you are battling a chronic neurodegenerative disease. It never occurred to me that inflammation could be another major cause of my depression until I experienced it for myself after getting sick from Lyme disease.

After about 10 years into the illness, a doctor told me that I had mast cell activation disorder (MCAD) induced by Lyme disease and mold toxicity. MCAD is a condition whereby the body releases an excessive amount of histamine from mast cells, which are a type of immune cell. The histamine causes widespread inflammation and can be caused by excessive exposure to dangerous toxins like mold and chronic infections, but it can also apparently be a genetic issue in some people or even caused by stress.

Researchers are finding MCAD to be a major contributing factor to many chronic conditions and illnesses: everything from depression to cancer to chronic fatigue syndrome. To learn more about MCAD, you may want to read Lawrence Afrin's book, *Never Bet Against Occam: Mast Cell Activation Disease and the Modern*

Epidemics of Chronic Illness and Medical Complexity. The book is targeted to medical practitioners but if you are science-oriented, you may find it interesting.

Both natural remedies and medications can be used to treat inflammation caused by oxidative stress and MCAD. Ketotifen is one of these. It is a compounded antihistamine medication with a very low side effect profile. Clark's Pharmacy in Washington is one pharmacy that makes this superb medication. My doctor gave me ketotifen for MCAD and literally overnight, my symptoms of Lyme and mold toxicity-induced MCAD were dramatically reduced, including the depression. Within a few days, I was a new person: happier, in less pain, and much more energetic.

What I like about ketotifen is that it is profoundly effective and, unlike other commonly known antihistamines like Benadryl, isn't anticholinergic; that is, it doesn't block the action of the neurotransmitter acetylcholine in the central and peripheral nervous system. Some antihistamines do this, and it is why drugs like Benadryl have been associated with Alzheimer's and memory loss, since acetylcholine plays a vital role in memory and cognition. On that note, be judicious when taking over-the-counter medications, because they are not necessarily safer than prescription drugs!

One natural antihistamine that may be effective for treating depression caused by MCAD is quercetin, a flavonoid antioxidant that's found in many plant foods. Diamine oxidase, an enzyme that's involved in the metabolism and inactivation of histamine, may also be helpful.

In addition, two natural substances that may help to reduce depression caused by inflammation are omega-3 essential fatty acids and curcumin. Both of these have been widely studied for their powerful anti-inflammatory properties.

Curcumin is a compound in the spice turmeric and has also been shown to be helpful for reducing histamine. You can purchase it over-the-counter and online. I recommend choosing a product that has a reputation for effectiveness, since curcumin can be difficult to absorb and not every curcumin product is bioavailable to the body.

Finally, perhaps the most effective thing that you can do to reduce inflammation in your brain and the rest of your body is to maintain an anti-inflammatory diet and reduce your stress levels. I have also found the brain system retraining programs, which I first shared about in Chapter Two, to be very powerful for reducing inflammation.

Infections as a Major Cause of Depression

All of us have pathogenic microbes in our bodies; everything from bacteria, to viruses, yeast, molds and parasites. Not all of us are sick from these microbes, as a healthy body will contain their numbers. However, if you are under stress, or your immune system becomes compromised by other factors, they can begin to reproduce in your body and cause disease.

A surprising number of us today battle chronic infections from microbes. Unbeknownst to many of us, they can cause a wide variety of symptoms, ranging from chronic fatigue to headaches, skin conditions, gut and cognitive problems, and, you guessed it—depression.

Microbes live in the central nervous system, brain, bloodstream, gastrointestinal tract, and just about every organ and tissue of the body. They can damage the brain and nervous system, gut and other parts of the body, and they release toxins that promote systemic inflammation, and consequently, depression. By now you've probably guessed that inflammation and depression are synonymous, right? Well, not always, but often, yes!

As I can personally attest, most people with chronic Lyme disease, which is caused by microbes that infect primarily the neurological and cardiovascular systems— battle depression and/or anxiety. The depression that microbes cause can be quite severe. This is because they damage or cause dysfunction in the brain, gut and other organs, and trigger widespread inflammation, which results in physiological depression.

Yet many people with chronic, low-grade infections often remain undiagnosed and unaware that they are harboring a plethora of pathogenic microbes, because current lab testing methods for pathogenic microbes are inadequate and symptoms of infection can mimic those of many other conditions. What's more, most conventionally trained doctors aren't trained to recognize these microbes, and tests haven't even yet been developed to detect the many species and strains of pathogenic microbes that are now in the environment and making people sick. Just because you have a negative lab test, doesn't mean you aren't harboring some pathogenic creatures somewhere in your body that are wreaking havoc!

The fact that pathogens can cause depression has been established by many studies, and doctors' experiences with their patients. For instance, a report from Stony Brook University states, "An analysis of 28 studies found a link between viruses and depression. These included the Borna disease virus (BDV), the herpes virus responsible for cold sores, varicella zoster virus, which causes chicken pox and Epstein-Barr virus, which causes glandular fever."[xxix]

Some examples of other common pathogenic microbes that cause depression include: *Borrelia, Babesia* and *Bartonella,* all of which are found in chronic Lyme disease. Many other types of parasites, bacteria and viruses can also cause it.

Mold and yeast infections such as those caused by *Candida albicans* are other major culprits. It is beyond the scope of this book to list every type of pathogenic organism that can affect your mood and wellbeing, so I highly recommend visiting an integrative medical doctor or naturopath, who uses an outside-the-box testing device or method to discover whether pathogens are making you sick or sad!

Two popular diagnostic devices used by integrative doctors include the ZYTO and ASYRA. Many non-conventional doctors now use these devices to test their patients for infections, as well as for many other things. They are computerized galvanic skin response devices that simply involve you placing your hand on a cradle, while a computer scans your body. They are a simple, non-invasive, and fast method for detecting problems in the body. Health care practitioners who are skilled in the use of these devices can detect a wide variety of pathogenic microbes that conventional lab tests will miss.

Other practitioners use muscle testing to find out whether the body is harboring a pathogenic infection that is affecting your mental health. Every skeletal muscle in your body is attached to or associated with your autonomic nervous system (ANS), which is responsible for the "automatic" functions of your body, like blood pressure, breathing, heart rate, digestion, and so on. If something is stressing your ANS, it will also cause momentary distress in, or a weakening of your skeletal muscles. So you can essentially "ask" your ANS questions by testing your body's muscle response to a variety of stressors, including pathogenic infections. Your ANS will respond by causing either a strengthening or weakening of the muscles in your body. Muscle testing, by itself, shouldn't usually be used as a standalone diagnostic tool, but when combined with other testing methods like lab tests and bioenergetic devices, it can help to confirm a diagnosis. For more information on muscle testing, see Dr. Cowden's and my book, *BioEnergetic Tools for Wellness*. Here, we also share some powerful tools in energy medicine for healing from depression, in addition to the solutions that I provide here.

Microbes cause depression through a variety of mechanisms, which may include, but are not limited to: inflaming the gut, brain and neurological system; disrupting hormonal function, and causing imbalances in many of the chemicals involved in mood, including multiple neurotransmitters. They also tend to affect the health of the gastrointestinal tract, where many neurotransmitters and mood-promoting probiotic bacteria are made.

Also, in neurological diseases like Lyme, the body can become overloaded by toxins generated by the pathogens, such as ammonia, in addition to toxins from the environment. Then, when the organs of elimination, especially the liver, become overloaded trying to process these toxins, this too, can result in depression. This is because liver health is also intimately linked to mental health.

For this reason, you may find it beneficial to do detoxification therapies on a regular basis, to help your body eliminate any toxins that are generated by pathogenic organisms. Many therapies out there are beneficial for this. These include, but aren't limited to: coffee enemas, ionic footbaths, castor oil packs over the liver, body brushing, rebounding, sauna therapy, exercise, liver flushes, massage, and taking homeopathic detoxification remedies such as those by Pekana and NutraMedix. These are just a few of the tools that integrative doctors recommend, to facilitate toxin removal through the liver, gallbladder, kidneys, skin and lymphatic system.

It is beyond the scope of this book to describe each of these tools in-depth, but you can learn about simple strategies for detoxifying your body and home of environmental contaminants, including pathogenic or microbial toxins, in Dr. Cowden's and my book, *Create a Toxin-Free Body or Home...Starting Today.*

Treatment for chronic infections can be as simple and straightforward as a two-week course of an herbal or homeopathic remedy, or months to years of treatment using herbs, essential oils, antimicrobial drugs, or oxidative therapies, which includes things like intravenous ozone. The type of medicine that you'll need will depend on the degree and types of infections that you have.

If you have a myriad of undiagnosed symptoms and find that changing your diet and taking nutritional supplements, and doing the other strategies described throughout this book doesn't seem to help much, consider that you may be battling chronic infections. These infections, just like environmental toxins, readily get into our bodies via the food, water, soil and air. They are prolific in the environment. Even if you aren't highly symptomatic, it is worthwhile to do a bioenergetic test with a practitioner who uses a ZYTO or ASYRA device, along with advanced lab testing and perhaps muscle testing, to find out whether pathogenic microbes are affecting you. You may be very surprised at what you find!

The Role of Gut Health in Mental Wellness

In recent years, researchers have been investigating what's called the "gut-brain" axis, which is all about how brain health affects the gut, and vice versa. I've already described one way in which leaky gut syndrome causes depression: by causing food particles to leak through damaged walls of the GI tract; specifically, the small intestine, where they enter the bloodstream and cause systemic inflammation. In addition, the type and number of beneficial bacteria that you have in your gut play an important role in your mood, as well as your immune function.

For instance, a 2016 study, the results of which were published in *Trends in Neurosciences,* found that the following probiotics (or beneficial bacteria) substantially reduced depression in a number of people:[xxx]

- Bifidobacterium bifidum
- Bifidobacterium lactis
- Lactobacillus acidophilus
- Lactobacillus brevis
- Lactobacillus casei
- Lactobacillus salivarius
- Lactococcus lactis

An article published on *MentalHealthDaily.com* entitled, "10 Best Probiotics For Depression & Anxiety: Gut-Brain Axis Modification" cites the following as the most helpful probiotics for mood regulation, according to animal studies. However, the 10th one on the list here is what's called a prebiotic, which is a plant fiber that nourishes the good bacteria that are already in the bowel or colon. While probiotics introduce good bacteria into your gut, prebiotics act as a fertilizer for the good bacteria that are already there.

The following pre and probiotics may help you to rebuild your gut, and in so doing, positively affect your mind and emotions. They include:

- Bifidobacterium longum
- Lactobacillus rhamnosus
- Lactobacillus helveticus
- Lactobacillus plantarum
- Bifidobacterium animalis
- Lactobacillus casei
- Bifidobacterium infantis
- Bifidobacterium breve
- Lactobacillus acidophilus
- Transgalactooligosaccharides

To find a probiotic supplement that will optimally enhance your mood and wellbeing, choose a product that has a high number of any of the above-mentioned multiple bacterial species. Ideally, also look for scientific research and clinical evidence to ascertain that product's effectiveness.

One product line that I like is that from Garden of Life (GoL), which contains a wide variety of live probiotic species that are guaranteed to arrive at their final destination alive. This is important, as many probiotic products that are on the market have been found in random testing to be completely ineffective.

For more information, see : www.GardenofLife.com.

Another great way to fill your gut with mood-promoting probiotics, or beneficial bacteria, is to consume fermented foods on a regular basis. Fermented foods often contain more types of beneficial bacteria than probiotic supplements and can be a helpful digestive aid.

Some popular fermented foods include: kombucha, kimchi, beet kvass, sauerkraut, and juices from fermented vegetables. You can also make your own fermented foods at home, which involves little more than soaking vegetables in a closed container for 48 hours with a little salt, and whey or starter culture. For easy instructions on how to make probiotic foods, and to purchase probiotic food starter kits, see: CulturesforHealth.com.

Gut health is vital for mental, emotional and physical wellbeing. For most people, healing the gut is multifactorial process that involves not just taking probiotics and removing gastrointestinal infections, but also healing a leaky gut and damaged stomach lining. In addition, it involves avoiding toxic, conventionally processed food.

Many natural substances heal and soothe a damaged gut. Among the most popular of these are: aloe vera, slippery elm, glutamine and marshmallow root. A product called Restore has also been shown to heal leaky gut, and while it's a bit pricey at around $50 for a month's supply, some doctors and other practitioners that I know have had great success in healing their patients' guts with it. For more information, see: Restore4Life.com.

For more in-depth information on healing the gut, an excellent resource is the book, *Gut and Psychology Syndrome: Natural Treatment for Autism, Dyspraxia, A.D.D., Dyslexia, A.D.H.D., Depression, and Schizophrenia* by Natasha Campbell-McBride, MD. Dr. Campbell-McBride has also developed a powerful diet for healing the gut, called the GAPS diet, which I mentioned earlier.

In summary, I encourage you to do further research on this topic, as you may be surprised to find that addressing and healing your gut with the right foods and supplements is a powerful tool that will bring you to the next level in your healing!

Mitochondrial Health

Other biological factors that affect mood and the mind include mitochondrial health and blood sugar balance. I will briefly share about these last two factors here, and you can do more research on each one on your own, as God leads you.

Your cells are made up of many components, including mitochondria, which are little organelles that are considered to be your cells' energy powerhouses, where all of their energy is produced. Much medical research of late has linked mitochondrial dysfunction and low energy to a multitude of health conditions, including depression.

For instance, one study found that people with depression had significantly fewer mitochondria, or energy producing organelles than those who weren't depressed.[xxxi] In another study, elderly women with good cognitive function were found to have greater numbers of mitochondria than those with poor cognitive function associated with depression.[xxxii]

Nutrients that facilitate mitochondrial health and provide energy to the cells include coenzyme Q10 and acetyl-L-carnitine. Both of these nutrients also have mood-enhancing properties, due to their ability to reduce oxidative stress and toxicity in the neurons and improve energy within the cells. Studies have shown CoQ10 levels to be significantly lower in people who are depressed or have chronic fatigue. Consequently, CoQ10 can improve symptoms of depression.[xxxiii]

Similarly, in another study on people with chronic depression, acetyl-L-carnitine was found to alleviate depression.[xxxiv] EASE

Therefore, you may want to ask your doctor if you could benefit from taking these vital mitochondria-supportive nutrients. They also support many other processes in the body, including heart health and energy production.

Another way to jumpstart your mitochondrial function is to get morning sunshine! Neurosurgeon Jack Kruse, MD, has found that bathing the skin in morning sunshine dramatically improves mitochondrial function, and with that, the cells' energy.[xxxv]

The Role of Insulin Resistance and Proper Blood Sugar
Balance

Over half of the US population is insulin resistant and has either pre-diabetes or diabetes.[xxxvi] Insulin resistance is a condition in which the cells become resistant to the effects of insulin, a hormone that's used by the body to deliver glucose into the cells, which the cells use for energy. Insulin resistance is incredibly common nowadays due to environmental toxicity, chronic infections, the Standard American Diet (SAD), which is high in carbohydrates, and stress. This means that many of us are hypoglycemic, pre-diabetic or even diabetic, as these are the outcomes of long-term insulin resistance.

Correcting insulin resistance and even some cases of type 2 diabetes can be as simple as adopting a low-carbohydrate and/or low-glycemic load diet. There are many books and resources on low carbohydrate and low glycemic load diets, such as the ketogenic diet. If you know that you are insulin resistant or have gained weight in recent years despite a healthy diet, it's worthwhile to consider adopting a low-carbohydrate diet and/or taking other steps to improve your blood sugar balance.

For instance, the natural supplements chromium and cinnamon have been shown to help the body uptake glucose into the cells and prevent insulin resistance. Regular exercise also lowers and prevents insulin resistance.

Insulin resistance is dangerous because it can lead to diabetes, heart disease, and other serious health conditions, including depression. In one study, patients who were treated with the insulin-sensitizing drug pioglitazone had less depression than those who weren't given the drug.[xxxvii] Evidence suggests that another drug that's commonly given to diabetics, called metformin, may positively influence mood, as well.[xxxviii]

If you aren't diabetic though, there are less toxic ways to improve the functioning of insulin in your body, such as through a low-carb diet, eating smaller meals, exercising, and taking nutrients that support healthy blood sugar regulation.

Studies show that for optimal health, your fasting glucose levels should be between 70 and 85 mg/dL, and two hours after a meal, should not exceed 120 mg/dL. If your blood sugar is higher than that, you are probably battling some degree of insulin resistance and should consider making some changes to your diet and/or exercise program. You can monitor your blood glucose by purchasing a glucometer and blood sugar testing strips from Wal-Mart or your local pharmacy. It's simple to do and a worthwhile tool for preventing diabetes, which has become rampant in the United States.

I don't mean to sound glum about all this, but the world in which we live today is quite different from the one that our grandparents or even parents grew up in. Diabetes, heart disease, cancer, metabolic syndrome, chronic neurological diseases and depression are epidemic, due to the fast-paced, stressful and toxic world in which we live.

Thankfully though, God has given us tools, including His Spirit, to help us heal our bodies from the onslaught of environmental toxins, so you don't have to be a victim of your environment! By asking Him to lead you in your wellness journey, you can be well equipped to overcome depression, or whatever health issues you battle. His Spirit is greater than all things, including the environment, and the degree to which we live out of His Spirit, is the degree to which I believe we will be unaffected by the environment.

That said, I encourage you not to disregard the natural laws that God has created for your wellbeing. He didn't create you to ingest toxic chemicals or fake, factory-made food. While you can't avoid all of these things completely, I believe that you will feel your best when you consume food in its natural state, take nutritional supplements as needed, and seek to detoxify and avoid those toxins that can make you ill, as much as possible.

At the same time, you don't need to live in fear and hopelessness, believing that the problems you face are just too great for Him to overcome. Nothing is too hard for God! He is more powerful than the environment, the devil and your flesh, and He can do in your life exceedingly, abundantly, above and beyond all that you ask or think!

Chapter Thirteen

Put Together a Wellness Plan

If you're feeling overwhelmed by now by all of the information that I've shared with you, please don't. You don't have to do everything that I've suggested here, or even all at once. Be led by God, your gut and what seems do-able for you right now. Do what most leaps out at you here, or what most excited you as you read this book. Chances are, those things are keys to your freedom.

In reality, there is only one major key to overcoming depression. That key will unlock every other door that you'll need to walk through to get well, and that is, your relationship with God! Therefore, if there is just one message that I hope you'll receive from this entire book, it is that you only need to do one thing to begin, and that is to spend time with the One who loves you richly and deeply, more than any other human or creature in the world. He has your best interests at heart, He's rooting for you, and He will help you to heal and overcome your battle with depression, disease or whatever it might be. His absolute will is for you to be well!

God once told me that it was more important that I trust Him than do everything right. Psalm 147:10-11 says, "He does not delight in the strength (military power) of the horse, nor does He take pleasure in the legs (strength) of a man. The Lord favors those who fear and worship Him [with awe-inspired reverence and obedience], Those who wait for His mercy and loving kindness."

I don't know about you, but that thought gives me great comfort. It means that God's hand isn't moved because we do all the right things; indeed, performance orientation and perfectionism are two things that make many of us depressed in the first place! His hand is moved because we turn our eyes to Him and simply say, "I can't do this, but you can, and I trust and believe that You will." Even if our emotions don't line up with our choice, we can say this and embrace these words wholeheartedly.

God simply wants a relationship with you. He wants you to come to Him with an attitude of positive expectation, gratitude and honor, but any work that He does in you to change and heal you will come about as a byproduct of your relationship with Him, not because you strive to do everything right.

As Oswald Chambers once said in his famous book, *My Utmost for His Highest,* relationship with God is about "trusting, rather than trying; surrendering, rather than striving" (paraphrased). This may be easier said than done, but yet less difficult than we make it out to be, because the more we know God, the more we will be able to choose to trust and surrender to Him, from the depths of our heart.

Your time with God doesn't have to involve a "to-do" checklist, unless of course, a checklist helps you. Just come to Him as you are. Praise and worship Him with a song or two one day. Meditate on, or "do" a healing Scripture the next. Talk to Him and ask Him to speak to you, and then journal His response to you. Or just sit in His presence and let Him love you. Don't get religious about it; just go to Him as a friend, son or daughter, and use the suggestions provided throughout this book as a roadmap to help get you started or to further define that relationship.

The other tools described throughout this book have been powerful for helping many people to recover from depression, but your relationship with God is the one thing that will enable you to live in all the fullness and richness of the life that He intends for you. He is the way, the truth and the life (John 14:6); the Alpha and the Omega, the First and the Last, the Beginning and the End of all things. (Revelation 22:13) You were created for relationship with Him, so you live, thrive and become whole only when your spirit is connected to His. In Him, you live and move and have your being. (Acts 17:28). These are eternal truths, and the more that you understand them, the more fully you will live in His love, and in the fullness of the health, joy and abundance that He's intended for you.

Beyond your relationship with God, I encourage you to ask Him about what areas of your life He wants you to focus on to get well. His Spirit alone can heal you, but He may want to use a few tools in the natural realm to help you along. Maybe it's a dietary or lifestyle change, making new friends, or taking some brain healing supplements. Maybe it's a lot of what I share in this book, but not all at once. And maybe it's something that I haven't even mentioned in this book, and which He has brought to your mind as you've read this.

If you aren't sure what God is leading you to do, allow me to suggest a way to prioritize the solutions presented throughout this book. Let these insights simply be a guide, or food for thought, at the same time that you realize that there may be other ways for you to get to where you need to go.

In addition to focusing on your relationship with God, I encourage you to first consider your diet and the foods that you put into your body daily. The right food is fuel for your soul, brain and body, and can powerfully influence your mood, in most cases, more than any supplement or medication.

God designed our bodies to thrive on natural, chemical-free foods that are similar to, or exactly as He created them in nature. If your diet has been poor for the most part, you may want to start off by making just a few changes, so you aren't overwhelmed. Research has shown dairy, sugar and grain products to be the most common food allergens and major culprits in depression, in addition to any artificial or chemically-laden foods, so you may want to start by first removing those things from your diet, as Holy Spirit leads.

Next, ask God what other factors may be causing or contributing to the depression and what you can do to cooperate with Him for your healing. If you aren't sure what He wants to say to you, consider what you already know and go from there.

For instance, if you are battling a chronic health issue or you know that depression runs in your family, you may find it beneficial to try some amino acids, vitamins or other nutrients to make up for what your brain and the rest of your body are not making or getting through your diet alone. Due to the toxic environment that we live in and our nutrient-depleted food supply, many of us have chemical imbalances and nutritional deficiencies that need to be addressed.

If you're a woman or man over 35, or you battle another chronic health condition, you may also find it important to work with a good integrative or natural medicine doctor, who can help you to get your hormones tested, and provide you with the right support to balance and heal them.

Once you adjust your diet and supplement regimen, you are likely to feel significantly better, and have the necessary motivation to make any other changes that you'll need to fully overcome depression, or simply live a fuller life. I can tell you from firsthand experience that I know how difficult it is to muster the motivation to do *anything* when your chemistry is "off"!

Once you give your brain and the rest of your body the nutrients that they need to function as God intended, you will most likely find it easier to do things like pray, work on healing any inner wounds, do a brain retraining program, go out and socialize and be a part of society; thrive in life-giving relationships, and take steps to fulfill your life's calling. Your human spirit, in cooperation with God's Spirit, is more powerful than your chemistry, or your flesh, but helping your soul and body along can sure help all three parts of you to function in greater harmony with one another!

Don't feel condemned because someone at church may have told you that you just need to have more faith for a miracle. Yes, God may heal you through a miracle, but He may also allow you to take supplements or hormones, or teach you how to renew your mind, as part of the healing process. Jesus paid for your healing on the Cross, but it may take time for you to learn how to appropriate that healing through His Spirit, who lives in you. And, for reasons we don't always understand, sometimes healing is a process and at times He will also use medicine, natural remedies, or other tools, to get you well. The key is to maintain your trust and faith in Him, not the tools. Besides, His Spirit makes all things supernatural, so whether your healing comes about as the result of a prayer or a supplement, know that anything that He leads you to do will be anointed and blessed by Him, and therefore, effective!

Creating a Sample Wellness Plan

Following I share my current wellness plan, to provide you with a brief example of what a happiness and health-promoting regimen looks like. This is to give you some idea about how to create your own, even though yours may look somewhat like mine, or completely different. Whatever you decide to do is between you and God.

In any case, I encourage you to create a list of goals and a schedule that includes the new things that you'll be doing in your life from week to week. Refer to the list and the schedule throughout the week so that you stay on track with your program. If you forget something, simply pick up and keep going. I encourage you to work with a friend on this; someone who can help you to stay accountable and encourage you if you forget to do things or want to give up at times (as we all do!). I also encourage you to work with a health care practitioner and/or trained minister or counselor, if possible.

Notice that I take a few supplements. I do this because I still need them. Lyme disease did a lot of damage to my body, and while God has healed me significantly, there are other areas in which He's still using tools in the natural realm to help me. I used to feel condemned for having to take natural medicine, because I thought that my faith should be enough to heal me, but I realize now that faith isn't the only factor in divine healing. Anyway, I believe God would want me to do what I can to be happy and healthy, right now. As long as I keep my trust and focus on Him, I think that this is what matters most.

In the meantime, God still uses me to supernaturally heal people of Lyme and other conditions, as He also uses me to educate others about how to know Him, and how they too can be healed using the natural resources that He's provided on the earth for our wellbeing.

After I awaken, the first thing that I do is meet with my beloved Heavenly Father, in my bed or my prayer closet. This sets the stage for the rest of my day. What I do with Him depends on the day. Sometimes, I will meditate upon a Scripture and ask Him to reveal the meaning to me. On other days, I will ask Him questions, listen for His voice, and then journal His responses to me. At other times, I will sing songs of praise and worship to Him or do some combination of all these things. Or, I will simply pray for others.

I try to spend at least an hour or two alone with Him every day, as well as acknowledge Him throughout the day. Occasionally, when I really need my spiritual tank to be filled, or I feel that He is calling me to spend more time with Him, I will spend entire days or weekends just soaking in His presence, which really recharges me.

After prayer, or sometimes even during my prayer time, I take my supplements and have breakfast. Sometimes, food and supplements can be a distraction, so I try to at least pray a little before I get out of bed and do anything else.

My breakfasts consist of organic turkey sausage and an almond flour tortilla, with pecan or another type of nut butter. I adopted this breakfast about a year ago, and it's my all-time favorite breakfast ever!

My list of morning mood-supportive supplements includes:

- Memory Works. This fantastic product contains nutrients that support dopamine, norepinephrine and energy production, as well as cognition. It has helped me to write books and function and gives my body a giant boost of "happy juice"! Memory Works contains L-tyrosine, choline, green tea extract, and L-carnitine, as well as a number of B-vitamins and a handful of other brain-supportive nutrients. To learn more, see: Xenesta.com.

- SAM-e, methyl B-12 and methyl-folate, which help my body to detoxify, as well as synthesize, utilize and break down neurotransmitters
- Transdermal choline, which the brain uses to make acetylcholine, a neurotransmitter that is responsible for memory and cognition, but which also promotes mood.
- Bio-identical thyroid hormone (T3), pregnenolone and progesterone, all of which support my mood, energy, sleep and other functions.
- Vitamin D-3, which indirectly supports my mood and healthy nervous system function.
- Omega 3 essential fatty acids from fish liver oil; quercetin, and a compounded medication called ketotifen, all of which reduce histamine and inflammation.
- Vitamin C and magnesium, both of which support a healthy stress response and adrenal gland function.

At night, I take a product called Kavinace, which contains 5-HTP, GABA and melatonin. The 5-HTP supports my mood, while the other two ingredients support my sleep. I also take CBN (cannabinol) for sleep at times, as well as CBD (cannabidiol) for muscle aches, both of which are components in cannabis that have non-psychotropic effects.

For lunch and dinner, I follow the principles outlined in this book, as well as *The Plant Paradox* diet. My diet consists of mostly non-starchy vegetables, low glycemic fruits such as berries and apricots, healthy oils and fats such as butter and coconut oil; pasture-raised animal protein and healthy nuts such as walnuts, pecans and macadamia nuts. This is a highly anti-inflammatory diet and ensures that I am able to function at my best.

Because I have a very full schedule, I don't make elaborate meals for lunch and dinner. I just throw most of my vegetables into a steamer or Instant Pot or put together a quick salad with a few leafy greens, some olives, goat cheese, artichokes, pine nuts and avocado. If you aren't a fan of green salads, consider adding some semi-exotic foods such as pine nuts, artichokes, pesto, olives, sun-dried tomatoes or capers to them, which makes them taste fantastic!

I bake or slow cook my meats in a Crock Pot or Instant Pot, which is an easy, healthy way to make easily digestible chicken, lamb, turkey, beef, eggs or fish.

Next, I try to spend at least an hour daily doing something relaxing, active or social, like going for a walk in the park, a swim in the pool, or out to coffee with a friend. I make it a priority to get out of the house at least once a week to see friends, or to do something fun. Because I work from home, it's very important for me to do this, or I end up feeling quite isolated after a while. We were made for fellowship with one another, and research has shown that people are generally happier and healthier when they are connected in life-giving relationships.

I try to combine my exercise, time spent in nature, and activities with friends, as much as possible. (It's my way of killing three birds with one stone)! If I can't do something fun during the week, I at least make sure that I have a little downtime daily, either to pray, read an uplifting book, watch an inspirational or fun television program, or talk to a friend on the phone as I exercise. This feeds my soul and spirit and helps me to rest and unwind.

I also periodically do infrared sauna therapy, ionic footbaths and coffee enemas, to remove environmental pollutants such as heavy metals, mold and pesticides from my body, all of which have been linked to depression. I also sometimes take toxin binders such as chlorella and zeolite. Detoxification is a practice that I believe that we all need to do regularly, due to the huge amount of toxins in the environment that we are all exposed to daily.

Finally, I pray for or minister to others periodically, either over the phone, in person, in public meetings or conferences, or as part of the bi-monthly prayer conference call group that I host once or twice a month with Bill. I sense God's joy when I do those things that He's called me to do, to build up and restore people, and it feeds my spirit, too.

While praying for people for 3-4 hours over the phone is challenging at times, it is also rewarding and I get excited when God sets people free from sickness and depression, or simply touches their hearts or lives in some other way. Doing ministry also helps to remind me of my identity in

God, and who He has created me to be, which is His mighty, precious, and powerful daughter!

What does your daily schedule look like? What might help you to do more of those things that you know will help you to break free from depression? If it's spending time with God, maybe you'll find that decorating your prayer closet with candles, or with wall plaques or prayer rugs that contain Scripture, or investing in some new praise and worship music, can help to inspire you and create an inviting prayer environment. Or perhaps finding a friend to go shopping or out on a walk with, taking a class, joining a social group, or making an effort to get out and about on a regular basis, will lift your spirits. I know it's hard to do these things when you don't feel well but make yourself do them! Inevitably, you'll find that you feel better because you made the effort.

Write down your goals, God's encouraging words to you, and His plans for your life in a journal, and then ask Him, day by day, how you can walk out your healing, the truth of who you are, and what He's created you to do and be, for your sake and that of the world that He's called you to impact for His Kingdom. Healing can be a process, but hopefully, the tools that I've presented throughout this book will help to shorten the runway for you. I wish that I had known years ago what I know today about how to walk out of depression, but I'm thankful that because of what I've learned, I can now help you.

Remember that it is God who fights for you and who works in you to "will and to do"! Now, simply look up, envision His loving eyes gazing down at you, and His strong, gentle hand reaching out for yours, as He says to you, "Come with Me, my child, for I have called you to walk in a life of freedom, abundance, joy, peace and everlasting love. Take My hand, and I will help you to live according to My Spirit, so that you may fulfill your years on this earth in health and prosperity of spirit, soul, and body, and in turn, set others free, too!" Amen, Jesus!

You can do this. You really, truly can. I have faith in you. And God does, too! May you be richly blessed in your healing journey.

Additional Reading and References

[i] Thomas J. Moore, AB1; Donald R. Mattison, MD, MS2. Adult Utilization of Psychiatric Drugs and Differences by Sex, Age, and Race. *JAMA Intern Med.* 2017;177(2):274-275 doi:10.1001/jamainternmed.2016.7507

[ii] Jackson Nakasawa, D. 2013. *The Last Best Cure.* New York, NY: Penguin Random House, LLC. Pp. xviii

[iii] Jackson Nakasawa, D. 2013. *The Last Best Cure.* New York, NY: Penguin Random House, LLC. Pp. 14-15.

[iv] Jackson Nakasawa, D. 2013. *The Last Best Cure.* New York, NY: Penguin Random House, LLC. Pp. 14-15. P. 37

[v] Hopper, A. 2014. *Wired for Healing.* Victoria, BC: The Dynamic Neural Retraining System. pp. 22-35

[vi] Clark, R. and Johnson, B. School of Healing and Impartation. *The Rock Church.* Castle Rock, Colorado. 2011.

[vii] Sandford, J. Loren and Mark Sandford. (2008) *Deliverance and Inner Healing.* Chosen Books, revised edition. Pp. 70-72

viii Sandford, J. Loren and Mark Sandford. (2008) *Deliverance and Inner Healing*. Chosen Books, revised edition. Pp. 64-69.

ix Mumtaz F1, Khan MI2, Zubair M3, Dehpour AR4. Neurobiology and consequences of social isolation stress in animal model-A comprehensive review. *Biomed Pharmacother.* 2018 Sep;105: 1205-1222. doi: 10.1016/j.biopha.2018.05.086. Epub 2018 Jun 22.

xx World Health Rankings. *World Life Expectancy.* Accessed on August 13, 2018 from: h worldlifeexpectancy.com/cause-of-death/alzheimers-dementia/by-country/ and worldlifeexpectancy.com/cause-of-death/parkinson-disease/by-country/.

xi Global Depression Statistics. Science Daily. July 26, 2011. ScienceDaily.com. Accessed on August 13, 2018 from: sciencedaily.com/releases/2011/07/110725202240.htm

xii Strasheim, C. (2016) *New Paradigms in Lyme Disease Treatment: 10 Top Doctors Reveal Healing Strategies that Work.* S. Lake Tahoe, CA: BioMed Publishing Group. Pp. 96-97.

[xiii] Strasheim, C. (2016) *New Paradigms in Lyme Disease Treatment: 10 Top Doctors Reveal Healing Strategies that Work*. S. Lake Tahoe, CA: BioMed Publishing Group. Pp. 96-97.

[xiv] Low levels of aluminum can lead to behavioral and morphological changes associated with Alzheimer's disease and age-related neurodegeneration. *Neurotoxicology*. 2016 Jan; 52:222-9. doi: 10.1016 /j.neuro.2015.12.002. Epub 2015 Dec 12.

[xv] Killin LO1,2,3, Starr JM1,2, Shiue IJ1,4, Russ TC5,6,7,8. Environmental risk factors for dementia: a systematic review. *BMC Geriatr*. 2016 Oct 12;16(1):175. *Biomed Pharmacother*. 2016 Oct;83:746-754.

[xvi] Maya S1, Prakash T2, Madhu KD1, Goli D1. Multifaceted effects of aluminum in neurodegenerative diseases: A review. *Biomed Pharmacotherapy*. 2016 Oct;83:746-754. doi: 10.1016/j.biopha.2016.07.035. Epub 2016 Jul 29.

Strasheim, C. (2016) *New Paradigms in Lyme Disease Treatment: 10 Top Doctors Reveal Healing Strategies that Work*. S. Lake Tahoe, CA: BioMed Publishing Group. Pp. 96-98.

[xviii] Sang-BaekKoh, Tae HuiKi, Seongho Min, Kyungsuk Lee, Dae Ryong Kanga, Jung RanChoi. Exposure to pesticide as a risk factor for depression: A population-based

longitudinal study in Korea. *NeuroToxicology*. Vol. 62, Sept. 2017, pp. 181-185

xix Strasheim, C. (2016) *New Paradigms in Lyme Disease Treatment: 10 Top Doctors Reveal Healing Strategies that Work*. S. Lake Tahoe, CA: BioMed Publishing Group. Pp. 96-98.

xx Davis DR1, Epp MD, Riordan HD. Changes in USDA food composition data for 43 garden crops, 1950 to 1999. *J Am Coll Nutr*. 2004 Dec;23(6):669-82.

xxi Strasheim, C. 2011 *Defeat Cancer: 15 Doctors of Integrative and Naturopathic Medicine Tell You How*. S. Lake Tahoe: BioMed Publishing Group. Pp. 335-336.

xxii Nancy L. Swanson 1, Andre Leu 2*, Jon Abrahamson 3 and Bradley Wallet. GENETICALLY ENGINEERED CROPS, GLYPHOSATE AND THE DETERIORATION OF HEALTH IN THE UNITED STATES OF AMERICA. *Journal of Organic Systems*. Vol. 9 Number 2.

xxiii Casella G1, Pozzi R2, Cigognetti M3, Bachetti F4, Torti G4, Cadei M3, Villanacci V3, Baldini V1, Bassotti G5. Mood disorders and non-celiac gluten sensitivity. *Minerva Gastroenterol Dietol*. 2017 Mar;63(1):32-37. doi: 10.23736/S1121-421X.16.02325-4. Epub 2016 Sep 20.

xxiv Northrup, C. 2010 *Women's Bodies, Women's Wisdom.* New York, NY: Bantam Books.

xxv Lebda MA1, Sadek KM2, El-Sayed YS3. Aspartame and Soft Drink-Mediated Neurotoxicity in Rats: Implication of Oxidative Stress, Apoptotic Signaling Pathways, Electrolytes and Hormonal Levels. *Metab Brain Dis.* 2017 Oct;32(5):1639-1647. doi: 10.1007/s11011-017-0052-y. Epub 2017 Jun 28.

xxvi Buser MC1, Scinicariello F2,1.J Clin Psychiatry. Cadmium, Lead, and Depressive Symptoms: Analysis of National Health and Nutrition Examination Survey 2011-2012. *Journal of Clinical Psychiatry.* 2017 May;78(5):e515-e521. doi: 10.4088/JCP.15m10383.

xxvii Chung MC1, Malatesta P, Bosquesi PL, Yamasaki PR, Santos JL, Vizioli EO. Advances in drug design based on the amino Acid approach: taurine analogues for the treatment of CNS diseases. *Pharmaceuticals* (Basel). 2012 Oct 23;5(10):1128-46.

xxviii Mercola, J. How to Get Your Vitamin D Within to Healthy Ranges. *Mercola.com.* Nov. 21, 2011. Accessed on September 13, 2017 from: articles.mercola.com/sites/articles/archive/2011/11/21/how-to-get-your-vitamin-d-to-healthy-ranges.aspx xxix Could depression be an INFECTIOUS DISEASE? Condition is caused by parasites, bacteria or virus and could be prevented with a jab, expert claims. *DailyMail.com.* Nov. 27, 2014. Accessed on September 13, 2017 from: www.dailymail.co.uk/health/article-2850645/Could-depression-INFECTIOUS-DISEASE-Condition-caused-parasites-bacteria-virus-prevented-jab-expert-claims.html.

xxx Sarkar, A. et al. Psychobiotics and the Manipulation of Bacteria–Gut–Brain Signals. *Trends in Neurosciences,* 39:11, 763-781. (2016). Accessed on
September 13, 2017 from:
www.cell.com/trends/neurosciences/fulltext/S0166-2236(16)30113-8.

xxxi Czarny P1, Wigner P2, Galecki P3, Sliwinski T4. The interplay between inflammation, oxidative stress, DNA damage, DNA repair and mitochondrial dysfunction in depression. *Prog Neuropsychopharmacol Biol Psychiatry.* 2017 Jun 29. pii: S0278-5846(16)30298-6. doi: 10.1016/j.pnpbp.2017.06.036. [Epub ahead of print]

xxxii Lee JW et al. Mitochondrial DNA copy number in peripheral blood is associated with cognitive function in apparently healthy elderly women. n *Chim Acta.* 2010 Apr 2;411(7-8):592-6. Epub 2010 Jan 28.

---

xxxiii Maes M, Mihaylova I, et al. Lower plasma coenzyme Q10 in depression: a marker for treatment resistance and chronic fatigue in depression and a risk factor to cardiovascular disorder in that illness. *Neuro Endocrinol Lett* 2009;30:462-9.

xxxiv Zanardi R, Smeraldi E. A double-blind, randomised, controlled clinical trial of acetyl-L-carnitine vs. amisulpride in the treatment of dysthymia. *Eur Neruopsychopharmacol* 2006;16:281-7.

xxxv Kruse, J. Time #11: Can you supplement sunlight? *JackKruse.com*. Accessed on August 23, 2018 from: jackkruse.com/time-10-can-you-supplement-sunlight/.

xxxvi Glatter, R. Half of adults in the US have diabetes or pre-diabetes, study finds. Sept. 8, 2015. *Forbes*. Accessed on Aug. 23, 2018 from: www.forbes.com/sites/robertglatter/2015/09/08/50-percent-of-adults-in-u-s-have-diabetes-or-pre-diabetes-study-finds/#1fd6378d47bd

xxxvii Kemp DE et al. Use of insulin sensitizers for the treatment of major depressive disorder: A pilot study of pioglitazone for major depression accompanied by abdominal obesity. *J Affect Disord*. 2011 Jul 20. [Epub ahead of print] xxxviii Ohaeri JU et al. Metabolic syndrome in severe mental disorders. *Metab Syndr Relat Disord.* 2011 Apr;9(2):91-8. Epub 2010 Oct 21

Chapter Three

Clark, R. (2012) *Supernatural Missions The Impact of the Supernatural on World Missions.* Apostolic Network of Global Awakening; 1st edition.

Clark, R. and B. Johnson. School of Healing and Impartation. The Rock Church. Castle Rock, Colorado. 2011.

FF Bosworth. (2008) *Christ the Healer.* Chosen Books; Revised edition.

Strasheim, C. (2010) *Healing Chronic Illness: By His Spirit, Through His Resources*

Chapter Four

Jakes, TD. (2013). *Let It Go: Forgive So You Can Be Forgiven.* Atria Books; Reprint edition

Sandford, JL and M. Sandford. (2008) *Deliverance and Inner Healing.* Chosen Books; Revised Edition.

Chapter Six

Cloud, H. and J. Townsend. (1992) *Boundaries: When to Say Yes, How to Say No to Take Control of Your Life.* Zondervan.

Strasheim, Connie. (2017). *Beyond a Glass of Milk and a Hot Bath: Advanced Sleep Solutions for People with Chronic Insomnia.*

Chapter Seven

Berkey water filters: BerkeyFilters.com

Cowden, L. and C. Strasheim. (2014) *Foods that Fit a Unique You.* ACIM Press.

Homemade Yogurt: www.MakeYourOwnYogurt.com.

Northrup, C. (2010) *Women's Bodies, Women's Wisdom (Revised Edition): Creating Physical and Emotional Health and Healing.* Bantam Books.

Strasheim, C. (2016) *New Paradigms in Lyme Disease Treatment: 10 Top Doctors Reveal Healing Strategies that Work.* S. Lake Tahoe: BioMed Publishing Group.

Strasheim, C. (2011). *Defeat Cancer: 15 Doctors of Integrative and Naturopathic Medicine Tell You How.*

Chapter 13 with Keith Scott-Mumby MD. S. Lake Tahoe: BioMed Publishing Group.

Chapter Eight

Brain entrainment devices: ClearMindCenter.com.

Frederick, B. (2017). *Recovery and Renewal: Your Essential Guide to Overcoming Dependency and Withdrawal from Sleeping Pills, Other Benzodiazepine Tranquillisers and Antidepressants.* RRW Publishing.

Cowden, L. and C. Strasheim. (2014). *BioEnergetic Tools for Wellness: How to Heal from Fatigue, Pain, Insomnia, Depression and Anxiety.*

Neurotransmitter and Hormone Testing Labs

Sabre Sciences (SabreSciences.com)
NeuroScience (WhyNeuroScience.com)
Pharmasan (Pharmasan.com)
BioHealth Diagnostics (BioHealthLab.com)
Strasheim, Connie. (2017). *Beyond a Glass of Milk and a Hot Bath: Advanced Sleep Solutions for People with Chronic Insomnia.*

Chapter Nine

To Find an Integrative Medical Doctor:

Academy for Comprehensive Integrative Medicine (ACIM): ACIMConnect.com
American College for Advancement in Medicine (ACAM): ACAM.org
The Institute for Functional Medicine: IFM.org.

Bowthorpe, J. (2011). *Stop the Thyroid Madness: A Patient Revolution Against Decades of Inferior Treatment.*

Kharrazian, D. (2010). *Why Do I Still Have Thyroid Symptoms? When My Lab Tests Are Normal: a Revolutionary Breakthrough in Understanding Hashimoto's Disease and Hypothyroidism.* Elephant Press.

Lam, M. (2012) *Adrenal Fatigue Syndrome - Reclaim Your Energy and Vitality with Clinically Proven Natural Programs.* Adrenal Institute Press.

Northrup, C. (2010) *Women's Bodies, Women's Wisdom (Revised Edition): Creating Physical and Emotional Health and Healing.* Bantam.

Chapter Ten

Afrin, L. (2016). *Never Bet Against Occam: Mast Cell Activation Disease and the Modern Epidemics of Chronic Illness and Medical Complexity.* Sisters Media, LLC; 1 edition.

Campbell-McBride, N. (2010). *Gut and Psychology Syndrome: Natural Treatment for Autism, Dyspraxia, A.D.D., Dyslexia, A.D.H.D., Depression, Schizophrenia*

Garden of Life probiotic and other products: GardenOfLife.com.
Key Pharmacy (for compounded ketotifen): www.keycompounding.com/.
Micronutrient testing: SpectraCell.com.
NutraMedix detoxification supplements: NutraMedix.com
Pekana detoxification supplements: Pekana.com.
ZYTO: www.ZYTO.com

Chapter Eleven

Cowden, L. and Strasheim, C.. (2014). *Create a Toxin-Free Body and Home: Starting Today.* ACIM Press.

Kavinace and Kavinace PM for sleep and mood: PureFormulas.com and NeuroScience Inc.com.

Memory Works for mood, mental function and energy: Xenestalife.com/connies/ (Note: I am a distributor of this product).

CPSIA information can be obtained
at www.ICGtesting.com
Printed in the USA
BVHW041950210820
586898BV00026B/293